NIPPLES!

Everything You Ever Wanted to Know
and a Little You Wish You Didn't

Jo Arquette

Table of Contents

Introduction

The day I told my wife I was interested in nipples—and not just her nipples but all nipples of the world—was day one of fourteen of me sleeping outside in the cold. Okay, while that's not entirely true, the icy stare she gave did make me feel chills for weeks. I might as well have taken my chances sleeping outside. Needless to say, it was a little more than a titty-bit nipply in the house after that epiphany. On the flip side, my own nipples could have cut diamonds with that frosty glance! And this only piqued my interest in nipples more!

Reaching adulthood as a heterosexual male (yes, I know how boring that sounds today) my early experiences were that the nipple was a challenging thing to interact with for various reasons. Hormones drove me into nervous exploration to bypass straps of protection but only if the holiest concession was granted: unfettered access to the breast.

The breast in its spherical form glides as it guides the hand aerodynamically to the destination of the nipple—earlier experiences were puzzling, devoid of what function is inherent once I reach this pinnacle. I mean, what happens next?!

While it was all incredibly memorable, and at times insatiably rousing, the inner workings of this majestic mountain I'd just climbed were utterly lost on me.

Like a dog catching up to a car wheel, I was along for the ride with someone else driving the car. I'm not really sure how the recipient of my amorous attention felt after snogging under a tree for three hours in a graveyard confessing our confused hormone-fueled lust for each other, but I began to ponder such things as I matured.

Later in life, when I realized that with age comes wisdom and endless quiet moments of reflection and yearning for youthful fancies, I began to understand the relevance of attaining a certain level and set of skills that went beyond simple snogging. Going for the gold in areola tweaking just wasn't going to cut the mustard!

I wanted to understand how the nipple functions in relation to the rest of the human anatomy: What is the role of the nipple during foreplay? Can there be too much, or too little, nipple stimulation? Is there a connection between orgasm and what happens to the nipple? Does this have anything to do with uterine contractions following birth and breastfeeding?

I had so many questions pass through my mind it was like all the blaster beams in *Star Wars* echoing through the star destroyer searching for Princess Leia. So I painstakingly sought all the nipple experts, nipple knowledge, and personal experience I could find on the topic and: Here it is! I refused to miss the mark every single time like a useless stormtrooper. This is the nipple information you are looking for!

What can one say about nipples that has not already been uttered in a men's locker room: A lot, in fact!

First, let's address the elephant in the room… Yes, they have nipples! Two rather large ones that function remarkably, shockingly like human breasts postpartum. And yes, they are quite large and hairy. I don't mean to ruin boobs for you, but let's appreciate their primary function of nurturing newborns. Hooray for boobies!

Back to the nips: everyone has nipples. Nipple knowledge is for everyone! Some may say it stands to reason that the nipple matches its owner in size, shape, number, and hairiness. So let's be honest, humans are no different from elephants in this regard: we all have nipples! Most mammals do. But what is their function? Why are these two circles stigmatized by certain societies and the rest of the boob area acceptable? What makes every nipple unique? Why do males and females have them while a select few of each species are born without even a simple set of nipples? Why are some people born with more than two nips? And why do they generally occur in pairs?

While two is usually considered better than one, there are actual biological reasons for the occurrence of two nipples per organism in the animal kingdom. Since humans are technically part of the animal kingdom, there are a few principles that still apply to their evolutionary roots as feral beasts. So let's begin with the basics: What the heck even are nipples? We're so glad that you asked…

Nipples! What Are They?

Imagine two fleshy orbs swimming beneath an ocean of silk. They exist just out of reach. Every second of every day, no matter the environment (work, home, on the train, etc.) these two mysterious circles are part of everyone's life. A glance in the morning mirror: nipples. A gust of wind that's too cold: nipples. "Ah, I spilled Diet Coke down my blouse!" And soon enough we're dabbing around the nipples because touching them in public seems too taboo.

How did society go from *National Geographic* nipples all the time to having these gems under lock and key constantly? Who regulates nipple exposure in the media and in daily life? Why can't we keep our nips out constantly? From the sensual to the prudential to the purely innocent way mothers feed their young, nipples have a complicated history for humankind. If we were all furry animals, nipples would be much less complicated… And if we're honest, much less sexy.

According to Dov Cohen, Ph.D. at the University of Illinois, cultural variation amongst humans worldwide may differ greatly based upon the level of food scarcity in conjunction with environmental harshness. In societies where protein-rich diets are lacking, breastmilk is not as nutritious and therefore must be eaten more frequently or the newborn risks death and deformity (Cohen, 2001).

Rigid sex roles proliferate these kinds of social structures to the point where practices such as polygamy abound. This may sound ideal until the beer money starts to run out and the supplies become low… But I digress. Men have many wives in these societies and women rear children among the females of the group. Children and their mothers share the same bed for a very long time after the birth of each child, hence the request for multiple women to share one man's bed.

The rigidity in childrearing (as a female responsibility alone) becomes a detriment to the entire population in this area. Women become tied to their children, literally by the breast. Men must hunt more often to feed the rest of the group. And daily life becomes a struggle. Boobs aplenty for the kids, and none are left over for fun time. All work and no play…

It is safe to say that in these types of communal living arrangements, the nips are generally bared and assigned a more functional purpose than a sexual one. Gender roles become polarized yet the breast is often acceptably on full display for all members of the group. Destigmatized breasts become both functional and decorative. A win-win for everyone!

Comparatively, Dr. Steven J. Heine (a Canadian psychologist with the UBC Department of Psychology) points out that "in cultures in which the environment is more benign and food is plentiful and more easily acquired, more androgynous gender roles are more likely to emerge," so this may explain the societal purpose of having two nipples regardless of being born male or female (Heine, 2016, p. 72). Androgyny makes everyone look physically more alike with a mix of feminine and masculine features in these cases.

Everyone is more equal in role and in physical appearance. It is further of note that in egalitarian societies, or the more industrialized and equal the members of a social group, the less likely a bra-free nipple is viewed as appropriate in public.

In essence, more civilized individuals are less likely to go shirtless. So let's "go Tarzan" in our next section: Nipples out!

Nipplegate: Modesty Culture

We're all fascinated by nipples. From a young age, as children are exploring their own existence, they all tweak their own nipples as an early discovery at some point. Be honest, if you have kids then you've surely seen this at some point. Maybe you've even secretly tweaked your own nips in private. Hey, no judgment here! It's innocent, it's endearing... Just keep it to yourself. Some may have even seen their older teenage brother continuing to behave in this way as a juvenile jokester for laughs. Others may shun the nipple to the point of banning feminine skin exposure altogether.

Consider the incident that would later be dubbed "Nipplegate" at the U.S. Super Bowl XXXVIII Halftime Show in Houston, Texas, in 2004. Janet Jackson and Justin Timberlake were scheduled to perform. The outfits both entertainers chose seemed relatively modest until Timberlake uttered the final line of the song "Rock Your Body": "Imma have you naked by the end of this song." And he did! As Timberlake pulled away part of Ms. Jackson's bustier, studded, silver nipple jewelry appeared, and with it, Ms. Jackson's luscious plum areola.

Whether Janet Jackson knew this was about to happen or not, whether she consented to some or all exposure, it is clear that she was embarrassed and upset. Nipples need consent! To view them is to attain the Holy Grail of an entire mountain of flesh. Entry into the nipple realm is a sacred blessing not to be taken lightly. Even a two-second glance could cost you dearly.

This two-second live television incident sparked so many Federal Communications Commission (FCC) censorship rules it's difficult to count them all! One lasting fallout is that live TV is now a few seconds behind the actual "live feed" so that censors can intercept any raunchy nudity or colorful language that my attempt to infiltrate any show attempting to be 'live' and spontaneous as it airs rather than be a pre-recorded bore.

Nips have consequences behind closed doors and in front of live audiences. One misstep and the fun has been ruined for every live TV performer following Nipplegate. Just ask Miley Cyrus. Nipplegate is likely why there was no "Twerk-gate."

It may seem admirable to avert the attention of young, impressionable minds away from such fleshy fiascos as a nip-slip, but the reality remains that in all actuality, nips will slip. No one is safe from the occasional side-boob, chilly nip, bikini calamity, or cup-runneth over in-your-face cleavage. Rather than keeping the cloth over poor Susie's eyes, let's instead educate ourselves in all things nipple! Knowledge is power!

Love Your Nips

Being a nipple owner is not always an easy task. Sometimes those twin clowns put on their party hats and put on a show in all the inappropriate, inopportune moments we wish they would remain calm. But there they go, writhing to attention in the most embarrassing ways and making us the life of the party when we were comfortable only being humble guests.

So why do nipples get hard? The answer is quite multi-faceted: much like the nipple itself. We'll cover this in-depth as the chapters progress.

And whether you own a twin set, an upper and a downer, an innie pair or outie pair, large, small, somewhere in between, ghost nip (no nip), or no matter how dark or light they are: Your nipples are as unique to you as your fingerprint.

Nipple shame is real. If they're hard all the time, ATTENTION! If they glow in the dark when you're trying to get it on, EMBARRASSMENT! If they are like dark eyesores, a bullseye for the eye, take heart. Take pride in the fact that there will never be another set of nipples quite like yours! Never be ashamed to bare those bad boys (or girls!) when appropriate (and legal). We don't want to have to bail you out of jail for public indecency, so make sure to check the laws wherever you are planning to unveil your cherry ice caps.

Chapter 1:

The Nipple in All Its Glory

Picture the sun: shining in all its radiance and warmth as its rays saturate your skin. Bask in the pleasure for a moment. Go on… Bask! But don't look directly at it! You can peek, you can steal glances, but looking directly at the sun is strictly forbidden if you don't want to lose an eye. The human nipple is like the sun in this regard. Social expectations implicitly state that the nipple has no place in most social settings… Even if we really, truly want to see it or show it.

There are exceptions to every rule: breastfeeding is one of the best reasons to reveal nipples in public. Even then, as the tiny human nurses, refrain from staring like a moth to the flame. This is dangerous and surely you'll erupt into a fiery inferno of consternation. Mamas tend to be tough, protective, and rightfully so. So please, do not attempt to engage the owner of these nipples. They're most likely minding their own business so it's best to mind yours! Instead, let's explore for ourselves (in private contemplation) what *is* a nipple???

What Makes a Nipple a Nipple?

General nipple knowledge is good to have on hand and *in* hand from time to time (wink wink). The nipple itself is comprised of several components that exist subdermally below the skin in addition to visible attributes like the areola and Montgomery tubercles that rest upon the peak of each fleshy mound.

Even in the rest of the animal kingdom, mammalian females and males of most species will have at least one set of two nipples. The main reason for this is to protect the proliferation of species: Always have a reserve breast full of milk. Baby's gotta eat!

Another reason for organisms having at least one set of nips is due to fetal development processes within the uterus, as we will explore shortly. A nipple's purpose is primarily set in species propagation: in sexual reproduction to stimulate the onset of labor and in nourishing the young. More on this later, but for now, let's explore the anatomy of a nipple, from base to summit.

Mammary glands run beneath the skin in an intricate labyrinth of parenchyma, stroma, and pectoralis major muscle in females. Parenchyma is functional tissue, in this case being used for the bodily function of lactation. These structures run parallel on both sides of the human chest but typically only present as two mound-shaped lactation systems located on the upper chest with the heart seated between. Possessing three breasts would leave nature struggling to find a fourth when the average human female is able to produce, and nutritionally sustain, only one offspring every year.

Three's a crowd, 'chestily' speaking.

Montgomery's tubercles or small, raised glands surrounding the areola, are present in both females and males. These sebaceous speed bumps serve the purpose of excreting antibacterial secretions responsible for protection against chest/breast infections since nipple ducts are considered an orifice, or opening into the body.

Generally speaking, most nipples have dimples that are rough and bumpy rather than smooth to the touch while the surrounding skin is more sleek. Aerolas, the pigmented area surrounding the nipple, are usually pink, reddish, or brown. The shape of these breasty bullseyes can vary from symmetrical circles to combinations of oval-circle targets for the eye. They do not always match! If you're searching for stars, you'll have to read on much further to find the section on pasties. And no, I'm not kidding. This is a legit non-fiction title about titty-toppers and we're leaving nothing to the imagination.

What about male mammaries? Worry not, we've got you covered.

Male nipples lack a functional purpose so their subdermal structure is less complex. Most male breast tissue is pectoralis major muscle and supportive fibro-adipose (fibrous support) tissue instead of fat deposits. Not that these nips are less important, they are glorious in their own right. They are just more adornment and playground for men than nursery and labor-lift-off buttons during pregnancy for women. Both male and female sets can be considered to have an erogenous purpose, so game on!

With their conical shape, nipples have a plentiful blood supply which allows them to elongate and stiffen when arousal is experienced. Arousal can be sexual. It can also be hormonally induced during breastfeeding to open milk ducts that facilitate milk flow.

Arousal can also include visual or tactile stimulation. In every instance, arousal means sensory stimulation of reticular formation fibers within the brain (American Psychological Association, 2022). Fluctuations in temperature also have the ability to constrict the fibrous muscles, or connective tissue, within the nipple structure (as in colder temperatures) or to relax these structures under warmer conditions. There is more to making the nipple erect than by sex or by touch alone: What complex nipples!

In short, the nipple becomes longer, and more malleable when warm. Silly putty nipple-stim sessions using body heat never sounded better. Breast play is more fun in the sun!

And remember that no matter what your spectacular set of milk duds looks like compared to what anyone else in the world may be sporting, your nips are as unique as you are. Appreciate who you are and the world will follow. Be beautifully, bravely, boob-tacularly you!

Primary Directive: Sustenance for Young

Full appreciation for those who are able and choose to breastfeed their children. Breastfeeding is an art form. It takes complete commitment, overcoming the first days of doubt (*is my milk even coming out???*) and it takes tenacity as well as ingenuity. Have you ever pumped breastmilk in a public bathroom stall because no lactation room was available? That's true talent. Anyone willing to put in that much time, dedication, and energy into nourishing a fully dependent tiny human being deserves massive respect!

The same muscles responsible for nipple tissue constriction play a part in breastfeeding and are located in the fourth intercostal space of the rib cage. Fifteen to twenty lactiferous ducts provide channels that run from outside the body, centered at the nipple tip, to beneath the breast tissue to finally end in the cavernous collection of lobules where milk is stored in lactating individuals.

Imagine a grapevine where the grapes are lobules and the vine itself is the lactiferous, or milk ducts that lead to the lactiferous sinus that pushes milk outside in a shower spray of marvelous milk. It's raining milk! Hallelujah!

Note that few beings are able to produce milk without repeated nipple abuse or hormone therapy so don't feel discouraged if you are unable to ever squeak even a tiny droplet out.

Back to the milk shower: Contrary to popular belief, milk does not leave the human nipple like it does the nipple of a bottle. More than 90% of human nipples contain between five and nine ductal orifices, comprised of peripheral and central ducts (Love and Barsky, 2004). There is more than one stream of milk that is activated in lactation. Unlike the single hole of a bottle nipple, the breast will release milk from several sinuses as the newborn suckles. Also, the ducts being used alternate until each lobule is empty only to be replenished again in time. What a let-down!

Letting down is the term used in breastfeeding that denotes the moment nerves in the breast signal for the nipple to release milk in a nursing parent or other lactating animal. This process is activated through suckling, by using a breast pump, or by hand-expressing milk. Hand expressing may make the lactating person feel akin to a pasture-fed bovine but it is sometimes necessary if the breasts become too full and begin to ache. Otherwise, that poor child may be getting an eyeful of the milky shower once let-down begins! It's an involuntary reaction, but it can get messy quickly!

If letdown produces an unruly flow, or the unoccupied breast becomes leaky, it is advised to press against the nipple using a hand, a towel, a nursing pad, or anything absorbent nearby to stave the flow. Think of holding pressure on a wound. This should limit any discomfort or embarrassment at inadvertently winning a wet t-shirt contest à la milk.

The feeling of letting down has been described as a tingling sensation that originates in the areola and becomes less intense as the sensation fans out into the surrounding fleshy breast tissue. This would be the lobules under the skin becoming less turgid. Consider it a spidey sense of feeling the web of milk leave the mammary glands.

Some people feel the sensation tickles and some describe it as being somewhat unpleasant. Further still, there are some lactating individuals who note a wave of nausea when their little one latches on to nurse. Whatever the sensation situation may be, a person being able to produce milk is one of the most magical side effects a pregnant person can experience once their baby is born.

Aside from sporting a dramatically enhanced rack built by increased pregnancy and postpartum hormones (which is another plus!), one of the most beautiful effects breastfeeding has is that it allows the mother to lose weight and begin to regain her pre-baby shape. Breastfeeding burns twice the amount of calories as were used during pregnancy! The action of nursing also stimulates the uterus to contract just after birth. Getting that uterus back to size ensures that everything which should be out of the womb is expelled. It can be a painful process to feel those contractions, but let's get mama healed!

For the newborn, breastfeeding creates a calm environment in which to bond with mom and explore their new world safely. It is no coincidence that the distance between breast and face is no more than a foot in length. This is about the same distance a newborn is able to see at birth. Making face-time even more important during those first weeks after the baby is born.

Bonding between parent and baby begins in the womb, but builds stronger once baby is able to see, smell, and touch mom skin-to-skin after birth. The first hour after the baby is born is considered the golden hour due to the importance of keeping mom and baby together to support this bond. There are biological, neurological, and physiological entities at work as mother and newborn reciprocate the same body warmth given off by mom's embrace. This helps calm the infant, regulate body temperature and heart rate. As the world bustles around them to clean up, support the pair who have just endured a near-year-long journey together. Bask in the love-glow with them.

You may notice how the newborn opens their mouth repeatedly. This indicates that baby is ready to learn how to eat. They've never known an empty tummy before, so let's get baby fed! Bottle or breast, making sure the infant is well-nourished is always best!

Nipples are super-important for babies and their moms especially in the beginning, but what do these bumpy orbs mean for men? Why are male children born with nipples if they will never be used for the same noble reason females might use theirs in their lifetime? Let's explore this more...

Man Nipples, What Are They Good For?

The fact that each nipple is basically, structurally the same while being wildly different only builds the excitement of finally being able to behold such splendor! Most male and female breast tissue contain one nipple and one areola on each side of the chest with ducts beginning to burrow into the body. Nerve endings abound radiating from the areola out and there is only one major muscle present, this is the pectoralis major.

For men, blind ducts end before more dense breast tissue, lobules, fatty deposits, mammary glands, and antilobular adipose or fat tissue abound beneath the skin. For men, it ends in blind ducts.

What else is new? Perhaps nips are the very reason men are from Mars and women supposedly hail from Venus. Developing the additional structures mentioned above proves the complexity of nipple function. So the question becomes: Can anything with nipples produce milk?

The simple answer is: no.

Male breast tissue does not maintain the structures necessary for the production of milk. Even if the hormones needed to begin lactation were introduced and fatty breast tissue formed, the factory for the ole milk machine is missing. Without milk ducts, lactiferous sinuses, mammary glands, and lobules, there is no milk to be had.

Instead, what may be mistaken for milk is really a byproduct of an underlying health issue. It is not true milk nor is it nutritional. It is typically lymphatic drainage and, in fact, you may need to get that checked out. Liver cirrhosis, hormone imbalance, tumors, and cancer can be legitimate reasons for these nipple secretions. So do everyone a favor, and please don't plop your nip in anyone's mouth. This leakage is not for human consumption! And honestly, it probably tastes terrible.

Sorry folks, Ben Stiller was wrong on this one... You cannot milk anything that has a nipple. Though you could still try.

Remarkable still is that there are a few male mammals that take on the role of nursing the young. Most notably are the Dayak bats found in Southeast Asia, along the Sunda Shelf where Borneo and Sumatra Island are located in Indonesia.

A type of flying fox, the male Dayak bat is known to produce milk though the reason for this remains unknown. Some explanations for lactation could be as complex as supporting their monogamous partner in nursing their offspring, or it could be as simple as ingesting pesticides. When the body breaks down these poisons, sometimes the effect is a mimicry of increased estrogen that produces more feminine attributes like growing breast tissue and producing a milk-like substance. Researchers are still trying to determine if the secretion is true milk or some other substance. Ew.

Phytoestrogens are an estrogen-like compound that stimulates milk production when ingested. These can be found when genetically-modified organisms (GMOs) like corn and soy are incorporated into the human diet. Or this phenomenon could be the culprit behind lactating male bats that ate some contaminated fruits and leaves producing the same effect.

Whatever the cause of nippy leakage, the result remains the same: males cannot truly lactate unless they possess the intricate internal system required for the milk to flow. I'm sorry to burst your busty bubble, but as compensation, you now have some useless knowledge to bestow upon your best friends over a beer. Lucky you!

Into Adulthood: a Playground

"Your body is a wonderland," or so says the John Mayer song. Sure, it seems counterintuitive to call such an adult act as lovemaking part of a "playground," but when everything is new, that is how it feels. The joy of discovery fueled by raging hormones can be all-encompassing. The passion, the ingenuity, the sights, the sounds, the smells titillating our very being to the core as we explore… It can be overwhelming.

It can be so overwhelming as to make our nipples stand on end. Stand up and salute!

But why does this happen, you may wonder. Several physiological changes occur during sexual arousal. One noticeable change is nipple erection. During sexual excitement, smooth muscles contract until the areolar skin grows wrinkled to become a close-knit clump of nerves. Bumpy like a basketball, this change also elevates the nipple until it protrudes outward away from the body. Consider it a signpost pointing the way.

Since millennia of evolution assigned humankind instructions to walk on two legs, sexual signals such as nipple erection became useful in mate selection. This statement is accurate primarily from an evolutionary standpoint alone; mind you, something that early humanoids would have found useful. Reading the nips to determine "go time" surely preceded more civilized social cues and sophisticated systems of verbal communication. It's not polite to search under skirts or inside trouser pockets to check if a mate is ready or willing.

Reading the nips, and more importantly your partner's lips, is definitely the much better, less criminal, way to determine if you're going to get lucky. No one's a neanderthal any longer so no excuses!

Nipple stimulation can be part of sexual foreplay or it can be ignored altogether. Nipples are not required for the act of sex, but they can help intensify the experience for both partners. Stimulating the nips releases the hormone oxytocin which is commonly known as the love hormone. Furthermore, the act of sucking can likewise release a heady mix of oxytocin and other endorphins. Experiencing rushes of oxytocin in the bloodstream has the euphoric power to strengthen bonds and ascribe pleasant memories of whatever is occurring during the rush.

Whether it be orgasm or the thrill of heavy petting, feeling oxytocin surge through your system can be incredibly pleasant. According to a 2006 study conducted by Levin and Meston, out of 301 participants, 81.5% of females and 51.9% of males felt that nipple stimulation was positively arousing during sex play. Of these participants, almost 8% found nipple play to be a turn-off. If this is to be an accurate representation of the human population, it would be safe to say that most people who have nipples find nipple stimulation arousing. Though it never hurts to ask first!

Nipple sensitivity seems to increase after puberty and peak throughout mid-to-late adulthood. Further study has shown that sensitivity wanes and increases dependent upon at what point within a menstrual cycle a female is with the most significant increase being observed within 24 hours after childbirth (Robinson and Short, 1977). It is believed that the rapid suckling of the nipple by the newborn just after birth serves as a catalyst for increased oxytocin and prolactin signaling the body to cease or delay ovulation and to produce milk in the mammary glands. An increase in sensitivity can also be seen during the midcycle period and at the onset of monthly menses.

That's all a lot of medical talk for something as simple as: Watch out because those nippies can be testy regardless of who they belong to! When in doubt, proceed with caution through discussion until the ice caps have melted and you can once again bathe in the silky-smooth waters of booby-bliss.

And Back to Pregnancy

Here: A random declaration by Charo from *The Surreal Life*, "Spooning leads to forking." It's true nevertheless! All that heavy petting and nipple stimulation leads right back to pregnancy. You can only play with fire for so long before you get burned… And it gets rather toasty rather quickly.

Nine months after the right (or wrong) timed hanky panky and you find yourself being a parent. It can be the most awe-inspiring or the most nerve-wracking time in a person's life. Whether you are the pregnant person or the support person, the goal is the same: Let's have a healthy family, baby and all! Or not; it's all up to you because I'm not raising anyone else's crotch goblins. I have my own.

Here's the skinny on growing that baby bump: the pregnant partner's nipples are along for the ride and will change rapidly during this rollercoaster full of hormonal ups and downs. So hang on! And put on your listening ears because the situation with the nipples changes frequently. Asky before touchy.

No two sets of pregnant nipples are alike. Some women find nipple stimulation intensely arousing during this period. Others may be blasé about it. And others still may find the experience completely nauseating. So grab a poncho while you're at it! You never know, it might be fun.

Bedroom play is about to become even trickier than finding a quiet spot to park your rusted jalopy to score a little tail as a teenager all while still making it home before curfew. It's time to get creative while you're creating your tiny miracle.

Endorphins and oxytocin likely landed you and your paramour in this predicament. Both hormones are released by, and reinforce strong emotions like, love. With about 20 kinds of endorphins surging through the human body at various times (while devouring something delicious, during sex, with hearty laughter, etc.), these neurotransmitters offer organic pain and stress relief. In short, they make you feel good so you want more. More sex equals a higher likelihood of sperm and egg meeting, making that chance encounter into an embryo.

Once that embryo sticks to the uterine wall, certain hormones will increase as a way to support the pregnancy: estrogen and progesterone galore! Oxytocin is usually present during pleasant times but will begin to have a greater impact on the course of the pregnancy. Granted, it's not an exact science, but nipple stimulation during the latter half of the third trimester (once your tiny turkey is more fully cooked) can bring on strong enough contractions to jumpstart labor.

A strong gush of oxytocin has the power to encourage contractions with a female orgasm. Orgasms and nipple stimulation release oxytocin and with that rush, the uterus and pelvic floor begin to contract. A surge intense enough, sustained long enough, can be all that is needed to tip the labor scale into full-blown, productive labor. Once that labor train pulls out of the station, there is no stopping the baby train from making its delivery.

So if you're looking for results, and you're both willing to re-enact the activities that likely landed you in the baby-way, as long as your doctor has cleared sex as okay, stim those nippies often. Everyday nipple stimulation and orgasm for the pregnant person is healthy for them, for you as a couple, for the pregnancy, and can lead to labor! The more, the merrier!

Feel-good love hormones abound! Endorphins and oxytocin will continue production throughout the pregnancy and are key players in the labor and delivery department. These two neurotransmitters are not pregnancy-exclusive (meaning that even non-pregnant people have the ability to produce oxytocin and endorphins). However, for this section, it should be noted that each plays a key part in labor and bonding. But how does this all tie into a nipple's purpose, you may ask. Good question. Read on!

Oxytocin is released during suckling of the nipple (i.e. nipple stimulation). Each nursing session brings about a new surge of connection, security, and love in the form of this heady hormone cocktail. Next, alveoli or hollow cavities in breast tissue that contain milk-secreting cells release colostrum (first milk) from the nipple's ductal orifices. This small amount of thick, sometimes yellow-hued liquid is not much in quantity but it packs all the necessary antibodies and nutrients newborns require in the first few days of life.

As the newborn grows, so does the amount of milk needed to sustain this new life. A mother's milk will come in within the first four to five days after giving birth. Her milk supply will continue to increase over the next weeks and months until the baby is weaned from the breast, which usually begins when baby food is introduced at around six months.

Prolactin, the hormone produced in the pituitary gland that is responsible for telling the mammary glands it is time to lactate occurs at normal levels in both males and females. Production amplifies during pregnancy and the postpartum period to around ten times the normal level naturally manufactured by non-gestating females. This baseline level for females happens to be twice as much as males normally produce. Welcome home baby, and mammoth mommy mammary mounds, too!

Those large breasts are not just for your viewing pleasure. They have a job to do! Be prepared for round-the-clock feedings and darkened areolas. That's right, even the rosiest nipples will grow darker (to a warm mocha or milk chocolate color) just before baby's delivery. Melanin, responsible for skin pigment, begins to increase production and self-tanning nipples is the result.

Note that nipples exposed to the sun during pregnancy will darken more dramatically. So be forewarned! Like all tans gradually disappear, this hyperpigmentation will fade with time after the baby is born. The purpose of pigmentation change is to benefit the baby in finding the mother's nipple after birth. Remember? Newborns have incredibly poor eyesight and need all the help they can get in finding that beautiful bullseye of nourishment.

Once breastfeeding is well-established, or a bottle of formula is introduced to baby, those *National-Geographic*-worthy milk saucers will reduce in size and return to their (mostly) original color. One amazing thing about the human body is its ability to adapt. Parenthood is a major adaptation for all parties involved so no pressure to return to a physical, mental, or emotional state that no longer exists, from the pre-baby era.

Congratulations! You're both parents now! Enjoy this fleeting time of nurturing new life, it goes by in the blink of an eye. You will one day regain unfettered access to those amazing Mount Everest mounds. Open and understanding communication goes a long way during the early years of having a child together. Give it grace and time; it's a big change for everybody!

Chapter 2:

As the Nipple Grows…

Now that we know what a nipple is, let's discover why the nipple is and even *how* the nipple is. How do those two chest accessories develop and why are they located where they are?

Let's discover the amazing process of growing nipples.

While we're at it, let's ask the important questions: why do some people grow more than two nipples? How does it happen that some are born with no nipples at all?

We're about to take a magical, mystical ride through the mammary ridge in all its nippy glory. Buckle up, buttercup!

Human Development: In Utero

It all begins in utero before a person is born. With 23 chromosomes donated from each parent in the form of gametes (sperm and egg) joining together to make a complete set of 46 genetically unique-to-you DNA genetic code, these blueprints tell certain cells to become fingers or organs or, you guessed it! Nipples!

Every embryo begins its journey through development as a 'female.' 'Female' is the default sex of all mammalian young in utero; ovaries descend as testes upon genetic signaling at a specific gestational point when it is time for the external genitals to form. In fact, mammary placodes are assigned nipple and breast tissue formation well before twenty weeks gestation when external sex can be determined more precisely via ultrasound. Nipples are evident before fetal viability is reached. All this means that because each embryo begins its developmental journey as the same sex, we are all gifted nipples.

Breast buds begin to form in both male and female fetuses along a "milk line" that runs vertically from armpit to groin in all mammalian animals. If you've seen the underside of a dog, cat, or pig (regardless of sex) you can see a distinct, parallel set of nipples—anywhere from four to eighteen nipples!—running along both sides of the animal's belly. Yet it is the presence of androgens during this embryonic stage of development (around week five) that determines the physical sex attributes of the fetus.

Genetically speaking, sex determination has already occurred at the time of conception with the egg contributing an X chromosome and the sperm contributing either an X or a Y chromosome. All of these examples are subject to genetic exceptions, however.

If estrogen increases, as is pre-programmed for an XX chromosome recipient, the fetus will remain female and breast tissue arrests development until puberty. If testosterone increases, as is destined for an XY chromosome recipient, the fetus will develop testes instead of ovaries, a penis instead of a clitoris, and will be considered male. These congruent tissue structures develop dependent upon genetic propensity, environmental factors, and are also influenced based on the amount and type of hormone present during critical developmental stages of the individual. Breast tissue will remain in a dormant state for both males and females until estrogen increases once again, if it ever does.

The interesting thing about hormones is that males and females alike produce both testosterone and estrogen. The main difference is the dominant level of which hormone is produced. This is the reason for more masculine or feminine secondary sexual characteristics such as facial hair growth (controlled by testosterone) or the presence of fatty breast tissue (controlled by estrogen). Primary sexual characteristics are the actual sexual reproductive organs like the penis, testicles, vagina, ovaries, and vulva.

So if you've ever noticed a woman sporting envy-inducing facial hair that you only wish you could emulate or a man with a rack better than your wife's, hormones almost always play a part. Let's normalize being human as normal! Happy humans are healthy humans, after all.

To recap: If a male who had previously never grown breasts starts to put on weight, begins hormone replacement therapy, or eats foods that mimic estrogen upon digestion (phytoestrogens) when the body detects this estrogen, it will form breast tissue around the nipple. So maybe that guy who wrote that book about Mars and Venus has it wrong, maybe we're all more similar than we realized and we're all just from planet Earth. Who knew?

Conclusively, males and females both have nipples because nipple development gestationally occurs just before sexual differentiation in humans and other mammalian animals.

May I also add that men should regularly check their breasts for lumps just like women are advised to do monthly? We'll touch on this later, but it never hurts to have a gentle reminder to man-handle your own mammaries because men can get breast cancer, too!

Budding Breasts

Ah, puberty... We all grow up one day. Puberty is not always the most fun, most exciting time in a person's life. Let's face it: It's awkward and knobby knees get in the way of bicycle handlebars and suddenly what was once a smooth ride becomes full of skinned knees... Adolescence is a mess! During this fleeting time in a child's life, many wondrous and potentially embarrassing changes occur within and to the male and female bodies.

Hair grows in places it never used to, body parts stand up demanding attention, and it all stinks. Literally! Body odor is one of the first signs that a child is going through this rite of passage. Antiperspirant deodorant is appropriate here. If only all of life's struggles could be solved with a little Rite Guard.

I jest, but when we talk about the nipples during puberty, it gets a bit awkward, and sometimes it gets a bit serious. Kids need guidance, they need reassurance. Kids, especially today, need to know that they are loved unconditionally. They need a safe home to voice their opinions and concerns.

They need to test their own voices because whether we adults are there or halfway around the globe, these kids will need their voices when they, too, become adults in this messed up world. Because let's face it, the real world isn't going to ever be able to offer them any sort of guarantee, not even about their safety.

But they'll grow up to be wieners, you may object! Wieners, winners, honestly who cares?? Even if they grow up being more empathetic, at least they'll be alive long enough to grow up, and they'll grow up knowing you're in their corner. Really, isn't that what parenthood is all about?

Time to get off my soapbox, public service announcement over. Don't get your titties in a twist.

Here, it's best to use factual, anatomically correct language when discussing "the talk" and body parts with children. Keep it age-appropriate, but keep it accurate. Knowing the anatomically correct language will help ensure that if someone touched your child's 'cookie,' you'll know they're upset about their missing dessert and not something far more heinous.

So, nipples. When males go through puberty, their nipples will begin to protrude a bit more from their chest wall no matter how flat their pecs had been previously. This is due to the sudden increase in hormones produced by their pituitary gland. Their body is trying to regulate the influx of hormone cocktails and growth instructions needed for gaining height and deepening their voices. Here come the growth spurts! As long as their diet remains by and large without phytoestrogens or GMO-ingredient, hyper-processed foods, their nipples will grow proportionately as the rest of their bodies grow instead of developing fatty breast tissue like females do. Male nipples will mature in congruence with the rest of their anatomy into adulthood.

Nipple growth in females is drastically different than in males during puberty.

It could be a real buzzkill when all summer you've been sporting the same one-piece bathing suit and suddenly by September, you're swimming with a t-shirt to cover your buds in the sun.

The science behind the summer shift in growing kids' bodies can only be explained by a combination of sunlight that contains vitamin D (needed for bone growth) in conjunction with it just being time to enter adolescence. Kids leave for summer vacation as children and return in the fall as gawky pre-teens. Don't worry kids, it happens, or has happened, to us all! You'll get through it, we promise.

Females will develop breast buds beneath their areolas. These can seem alarming at first because they feel like hard lumps and make the breast appear conical in shape beneath shirts that had once rested flat against the chest. Not to worry, these 'buds' are developing mammary glands and initiating the growth of the intricate ductwork that will one day enable them to breastfeed as women, when and if they are ready and choose to do so.

So break out the training bras and bring a lot of gentle understanding because as awkward as taking a child to try on their first bra can be, it's even more embarrassing for the child. And it's pretty uncomfortable, too.

The increased blood flow to the nipple area also heightens nipple sensitivity. Suffice it to say that this increased innervation can also signify that it's time to purchase pads and Midol for the onset of menstruation. Nipple and breast sensitivity is linked to increased hormone production of the estrogen and progesterone that are responsible for monthly cycle regulation. So once those buds start blooming, batten down the hatches and prepare for the deluge of adolescent angst about to come your way. God bless you.

Following the Milk Line

What is the milk line? Sure, it sounds like a factory for milk-making or milk delivery, but in all actuality, it is the layman's term for the mammary ridge. This parallel line down both sides of an organism's ventral or front half of the body, from underarm to groin, is mostly invisible in adults. This is where you will find nipples. In fact, this is the line seen in embryonic development that is easily identified as a thickened band of developing ectoderm (or skin). The number of nipples the organism will have is easily seen at this early gestational age. Once that embryo is fully developed, the mammary line disappears.

Enlarged cells become multilayered placodes that then morph into hillock buds and bulbs (like a plant taking root). From there, as the organism matures outside the womb, these branches grow deeper into the breast tissue during puberty.

Here's where it gets a little tricky. Nipple development along the mammary ridge can vary in lactiferous duct depth, the number of lobules that are able to produce milk, and level of functionality. While there could be eighteen nipples on a pig, not every one of those porky peaks will work at the same caliber as others along that same milk line. Not all nipples are created equal in this instance.

This can create runts in litters because there's just not enough milk to go around and everyone's fighting for the best nipple. If animals would be able to take turns then all littermates would be well-nourished. Sadly, this is just not the case in the animal kingdom (with the exception of humans… most of the time). Can't we all just get along?

Extra Nipples!

We examined how having multiple nipple sets occurs in utero when the species in question is meant to have more sets of nips than the standard two; we even discussed how bum nippies create undernourished runts.

It's now time to explore the world of extra nipples. These are the nips with no functionality whatsoever. These are for show.

Who doesn't love accessories? There are literally hundreds of thousands of stores out there that only sell accessories. They're so cute, they're so trendy. What else falls into the category of cute accessories? Extra nipples, that's what.

Accessory nipples can be found in roughly one to five percent of the human species. In theory, a person could have a supernumerary nipple hanging out right next to the baby factory because the milk line, or mammary ridge as it's officially known, (where these extra nipples develop) runs all the way from the groin up to the armpit. In actuality, the majority of polythelia—that's what the condition of having supernumerary nipples is called—presents as nipples along the torso.

It's not as uncommon a condition as you may think. Roughly one percent of women have supernumerary nips. That's still approximately 78 million people! The other four to five percent of affected individuals is male, so you can see that multiple nipples is found more often in males than in females. Nature doesn't always make the most sense, but we'll go with it.

Eutherian mammals, or animals including humans that require a placenta in utero to sustain fetal development until birth, sport nipples. Even most marsupials in this category have nipples, although the duck-billed platypus does not. There are absolutely no nipples to be found there! And they're venomous… So who knows what's going on with those wiley critters!

According to the American Museum of Natural History, the duck-billed platypus is one of the few species of mothers who lays eggs, has no nipples, but still manages to produce milk for its young by having it ooze directly out of its mammary glands, onto its fur. Once in the platypus's fur, the milk is then ingested by baby platypuses as if the fur were a teat, like sucking on a very furry straw. What strange, mixed-up little creatures… But they get the job done.

In the human population, the chance of a person being born with extra nipples is about 5 in 100. The opposite condition of having no nipples (like a platypus) is termed athelia. Having this condition is even rarer than having too many teats.

The most common cause of failure to develop nipples is Poland syndrome and it occurs in about 1 in 20,000 births (Watson, 2018). Here we are again at that crucial six weeks gestation when the mammary ridge is supposed to be super-visible. It's at this point that it is believed improper circulation causes Poland syndrome.

Ectodermal dysplasia and autosomal dominant inheritance genes may also be to blame for failure to develop nipples. These conditions affect males and females in about equal quantities, while Poland syndrome is typically seen more in males as researcher Stephanie Watson (2018) points out in her article on the subject. Not only do men have blind ducts, sometimes they have absolutely no ducts. That sucks!

Too many, or not enough nipples, can be cause for aesthetic concern, but have no fear! There are cosmetic ways to change your nipple situation no matter the category into which you fall.

Surgical removal of extra nipple and breast tissue may prove to be the correct route for you. Or you may choose to have nipple-esque appendages surgically constructed from other similar body tissues you possess (lips to nips anyone?). These would be purely ornamental because, regrettably, there is no way for even the best breast surgeons to reattach and create those tiny nerve-endings that would make your new nips as sensitive as if they'd been there your whole life. Sorry to burst your busty bubble.

Know that you are not alone in your state of supernumerary nipple(s). Actor Mark Whalberg, country singer Carrie Underwood, celebrity Zac Efron, and singer Harry Styles all sport more than two chest adornments. These celebrities have never let their supernumeraries stop them from success. Mark Whalberg and Harry Styles certainly take no issue in taking off their shirts for paparazzi to bask in the splendor that is their superlative stalagmites.

For the record, I totally get why Carrie Underwood never exposed hers. There are rules about that sort of thing purely based on Ms. Underwood being a woman. Sources say she even had her accessory nipple removed.

That's one way to go about getting rid of the elephant in the room, or in this case the nipple everyone knows about but you wish they wouldn't. It's almost as bad as having that dream where you walk in the room and everyone you know is there... And you're butt-naked. It may seem mortifying but at least the extra nipple situation has a solution. I don't know what to say if you suddenly find yourself naked somewhere in publc... Hopefully that just stays the stuff of nightmares.

Chapter 3:

Sensuality or Stigma

Now that I've piqued your interest about the possibility that a mammary mountain range that might be lurking beneath a person's shirt, I've got a question for you: What's sexier than a tiny chest tent in a wet t-shirt contest? Not much to be honest, but here we are imagining one anyway. Once the floodgates of imagination open, it's easy to get swept down a rabbit hole and suddenly we're swimming with Dolly Parton near islands in a stream, captivated by cones trapped beneath sopping wet cotton that clings.

What makes these two round mound ornaments so appealing? Perhaps the fact that the eye is drawn directly to the nipple is the correct answer. Or even from birth, newborns follow a biological, evolutionary urge to smell, seek, and look for the nipple in order to survive. The short answer is that humans are programmed to notice anything that seems out of place or suspicious. This involuntary response is a leftover survival instinct from our hunter-gatherer days.

While survival being directly related to the breast diminishes with age, there are biological reasons adults still seek the nipple. The health of a suitor or even subconscious determination of breeding excellence may be 'read' in the nipples. The better the nips, the better the genes, perhaps. Being able to determine a person's virginity also used to be deciphered by studying the nipple in the nude to see if any pregnancy-related changes had occurred.

Certain tribes keep this practice alive today out of tradition. In Nigeria, for instance, council elders will line up adolescent females from their village as they begin to come of age. The onset of menses or reaching a certain age signals it is time for this rite of passage to commence. While fallible in accuracy and seeming to dehumanize these young girls, practices like these are still revered in certain cultures.

We'll cover this more in-depth later, but for now, know that nipples tend to give away a few of the wearers' secrets: especially if you know what characteristics to look for in determining certain levels of health, maturity, or life experience. Even stolen glances have the potential to provide pertinent information about the nipple bearer. Perhaps, "Read my nips," instead of the usual "Read my lips" might catch on as the new catchphrase for when you mean business. No? Well it was worth a try.

From Purple Nurples to Pleasure

Red is the color of passion, love. Purple is passionate too, but it also signals bruising and pain. We're all for tweaking those nippies but no twisting, please! Unless specific instructions are given to do so, that is. Some like it rough.

An ample blood supply is necessary for the constriction and smooth release nipples endure in a day's work. Blood moves through the breast tissue, into the areolas and nipples during all hours of the day. It follows the central mammary artery otherwise known as the internal thoracic artery. After that, a mix of superficial and deep veins spread out to supply the rest of the breast with oxygenated blood to keep the tissue alive and perky. The blood is then filtered back to the heart to begin the entire process all over again.

All this rushing blood means increased sensitivity. The higher the arousal, the greater the blood flow, and the less pressure it may take to achieve the desired effect: pleasure. During sexual arousal, the nipple area becomes engorged with blood and with it, heat. Blood is hot! Did we mention that mammals (which includes humans) are warm-blooded? As body temperature increases, so does the sensitivity of the nerves within the tissue. So a little bit may go a lot further in terms of mutual satisfaction.

So while the purpose of a purple nurple may seem like a childhood prank, the science behind the pain it can cause is quite simple. Extra blood flow, enhanced sensitivity, too much torque, and voila! What could have been pleasure becomes intense pain. Some people can be so sadistic, which is okay if you're both into that sort of thing.

Now that we understand nipple blood flow, let's explore the pain or pleasure perception related to this ample appendage: the nipple nerves.

The Nerve

Some cups runneth over. While one may argue that having too much of a good thing is wonderful, others may tell a different tale. The entire male fantasy is generally built around a pair of perfect, perky, and rather LARGE breasts bouncing in slow-motion to the beat of some '80s rock anthem. Cue the *Baywatch* theme!

But most women who possess large breasts will tell you what a pain they can be. Running track in high school comes with its own crowd of raucous applause following you around the track as large breasts clap against the sternum with every hurtling stride. It's embarrassing at best and excruciatingly painful for the breast and back at worst.

Studies of breast innervation will side with the ladies. Longo, et al., found chronic nerve traction injury in individuals with large, heavy breasts (Zucca-Matthes, Urban, and Vallejo, 2016). It stands to reason that the smaller the breast, the more sensitive it (and the nipples) are.

Keep in mind that bigger is not always better.

On the other hand, breast tissue being super-sensitive can have its perks. There exists a phenomenon where females are able to reach orgasm through nipple stimulation alone. Tweaking the nipply bits in just the right accord has the uncanny ability to make some women sing!

Researchers Komisaruk, et al. (2011), discovered that the anatomy of the female orgasm does not only manifest in the vagina, clitoris, or cervical areas but can be activated during nipple stimulation, too. Specifically, it is noted that self-nipple-play triggers the genital sensory cortex. This discovery was surprising, but it supports a complex neurological understanding of female erogenous zones.

So whether you have or hold a pair of breasts, it is always important to remember that each chest is individual and worthy of attention no matter the cup size or appearance, as long as the adults involved emphatically consent to such attention, that is.

Nipples in the Closet

Afraid to bust those bad boys (or girls) out of their everyday attire? Don't be! Nipples are one of the most natural parts of the human body. It has been ascertained that there exist roughly nine different types of nipples. Maybe we'll even figure out what kind of twin peaks you're sporting. Let's dive in…

First, and most common, are the nipples that lift off the chest or protrude outward. These perky, pert peaks rise above no matter what gravity throws at them. When you think nipple, these are often the type that comes to mind. They're great for breastfeeding, making a rack out of that blouse, and keeping your wet t-shirt from sticking to your chest.

Next in line would be the flat nipple. These are the middle-man of the nipple world and offer very little in the way of tree-topping tenacity. Not that these flattops are lesser nipples because of their appearance, but the reality of the situation is that the further the nipple inverts into the chest, the more difficult a time the flattop-nip-owner will have in nursing their newborn.

This brings us to the third type of nipple: the inverted nipple. This stud enters the Upside Down as more an innie than an outie. Even the fourth set of nippies, the unilaterally inverted ones, make breastfeeding difficult because—though the areola does protrude—the area containing the milk ducts, the nipple itself, ducks back into the chest wall.

Halfway through our quest for nipple nuances, we move onto the fifth type of mammary mound-toper featuring the Montgomery glands. These spackled studs appear bumpy but are completely normal, especially if the nipple-owner is pregnant or nursing. For whatever evolutionary reason, these lumpy lactators allow nearly blind newborns to reach the breast as if they were reading braille. Being so new and able to scoot to the source of their sustenance is quite a commendable feat!

Now, we move onto the sixth type of nipple and this is where things get a bit hairy. Ah, the hairy nipple, the beastly breast: Why do they exist and how do we comb through to find all that perky glory? Moderate amounts of body hair sporadically appearing on the human body is a carry-over from our less attractive Neanderthal days when we were more true to being animals than intelligent human beings. The jury is still out about some modern specimens of *homo sapiens*.

Honestly, nipple hair is much more common than you may believe. Though it is generally associated with the male set of nips, females also have less prominent chest hairs (even ones that sprout from their areolas). It's normal, no one needs to pluck it to be perfect. Let's all be mature. If you feel it's personally necessary to manicure your own mammaries, waxing is the less painful option over shaving. It sounds counterintuitive but the truth is that waxing needs to be done less often and there is no razor burn afterward.

From the hairy chest, we move on to the puffy chest. These adornments melt into the surrounding breast tissue as both nipples and areolas protrude out and about, proud as a peacock to liftoff and strut into the public eye. Who could resist even a passing glance? Puffy nipples tend to be part of having new breasts (for males and females) during puberty when hormones go all wonky and we all wish we could just hide until adolescence ends. Word of advice, try to avoid glancing at underage ribcages. It's gross.

The last two kinds of nipples have already been discussed: extra nipples and nonexistent nips. Having too many or none at all can put a hindrance in anyone's plans regardless of sex. Imagine buying a bikini and having nothing to fill it with, nothing to keep the two tiny pieces of decorative cloth in place. Imagine the inverse of literally looking like you're about to feed a litter with all those extra nipples. That's so frustrating!

That's nine kinds of nipples in all: perky, flat, inverted, unilaterally inverted, bumpy, hairy, puffy, supernumerary, and ghost nips or no nips.

Nipples are not *only* made for nursing but having innies where outies are preferred for ease of use does complicate the process. Also, getting in that coveted supple nipple action could prove more arduous with inverted nipples. Every challenge has its victory and the rewards are many, so we encourage you to keep trying! You only truly fail if you quit.

Raisins in the Sun

My nips got chills, they're hard as diamonds… The tricky thing about nipples is that they can be both hard and soft, while simultaneously being either something you never think about or something you obsess over constantly like a hairy mole you've been trying to hide since grade school gym class. Maybe that's why Carrie Underwood had hers removed.

But what if you're somewhere in the middle and you just don't care who sees your nips in whatever state they decide to be in for that day? Well… You just wing it! Apricate those apricots like raisins in the sun!

Step out into the sunshine, nips first, and seize the day! But be sure to bring your sunscreen or those usually subdued ninjas will rise to the occasion, a blister in the sun.

Prevention is key here, but if you do find yourself with a double helping of chest raisins, wrinkled and enraged, one option for relief for this sensitive sunburn would be to use a soothing aloe balm. This miracle salve is usually a cool blue or an aloe green. Slather that stuff on generously. Leave no slice of meat-pie dry.

One amazingly magical thing about this stuff is that is tends to feel cooling even when the bottle is kept at room temperature. You can find it in the pharmacy section probably next to the sunscreen… Which is what we suggest you wear first. Tsk tsk.

Remember that nipples do darken when exposed to sunlight, especially if the person baring their nips makes more melanin (skin pigmentation, not to be confused with melatonin that makes someone sleepy). Someone who is pregnant may also find they have splotches of various light and dark spots on their skin and their nipples appear more deeply hued due to a combination of UV exposure and hormonal changes.

Hormones and melanin make a mean mix of hyperpigmentation that can create a total eclipse of the areolas for months. Rest assured that those painted peaks will revert to their original color eventually. No one is pregnant forever and tans gradually fade.

Chapter 4:

Are My Nipples Normal?

To everyone reading this book or sharing random pages between judgmental glances from onlookers over your shoulder in the bookstore (yeah, we see you!), the loud resounding answer to what everyone wants to know is: Yes! Your nipples are normal.

Everyone's nipples, or condition of having no nipples, is normal. Normal is honestly whatever you make it. There is no real "normal" or status quo. Whatever you've been led to believe about what makes a person valued or acceptable by societal standards can get thrown right out the window. Time to take out the trash! Better yet, let the trash take itself out.

Unload your heavy burdens about what the media tells you is beautiful, attractive, or attainable without a personal trainer and a meal plan the size of a grape. Each individual is perfect the way they are. The world should adjust its expectations. Differences in nipple appearance, breast size, shape, and having nippies or not makes no exception to this plan of acceptance. Rock those raisins with pride!

While we're in an egalitarian mode, here's another tidbit about the tittie area you should know: Male nipples and female nipples should be treated equally!

That's right! We're taking the hard stance that all nips should be censored or no nips should be. It's all or nothing so let's keep it equal. After all, 'equal' is how all humans began in the womb... Hence the reason behind (almost) everybody having nipples in the first place. We rest our case...

A word of caution, however. Personal beliefs are not law, but make sure that wherever you choose to unleash your fleshy beasts you won't be charged with public indecency or worse. What is considered a punishable offense differs widely across the globe so gain a thorough grasp of local laws wherever you go and be sure you know the possible ramifications of releasing your rowdy red raspberries. We don't have enough bail money if you make a miscalculated nip slip.

National Geographic: The Natural Nipple

Natural nipples, those as seen on the cover of old *National Geographic* magazines may seem shocking. There may even be a few shrewd prudes with gnarly attitudes who think the sharply detailed and sometimes graphic granite busts and other artwork in museums are too obscene for public display.

Be consoled, we are not those kinds of people.

Censor what your own children under your care view and consume, sure. But don't spoil it for the rest of us.

Granted, people of the world who grow up in societies where nudity is common see nothing wrong with living their lives *au natural,* as well. Living this way doesn't make these communities wrong or sinful. This is a fine example of how minding one's own business leads to deeper levels of happiness within the eye of the beholder and within those being spied upon by outsiders.

There is no need to 'fix' cultures until they reach Western standards. Colonization went out of style long ago. 'Normal' means different things to different people under different circumstances. Live and let live!

Now that our nippies have gone all hippie, know that frequently hugging trees while topless could irritate your titty-toppers. It's not recommended to make this a habit but in case you find yourself in need of a little nipple advice, keep reading to discover a few new ways to calm those tempestuous teats.

Common Nip Complaints

Dry, itchy, redness, soreness, and embarrassing discharge are all symptoms nip-owners cannot ignore. When those two miniature mountains start screaming for attention like a toddler in the middle of a packed mall on Christmas Eve, you certainly must give attention and take necessary care.

Sometimes the reason behind the rash is easy to discern. Rash guards are a wonderful solution to wind burn and chest chaffing as a result of long days on the beach. Don't let the friction of sand and surf set your nippies on fire! Catching a rash while trying to catch a wave is the exact opposite of being totally tubular. So when you've been rubbing your chest-roses against a surfboard all day and need more protection than sunscreen alone can provide, the answer is to wear a rash guard. These lightweight, synthetic shirts protect those sensitive party hats so you can continue the fun in the sun.

Treating those screamy, highbeam headlights when they're cracked and dry can be a nightmare. Relief is in sight! Moisturize, moisturize, moisturize! Lanolin nipple balm is not only recommended for nursing mothers, it is a moisturizing salve made from lamb oil that is found naturally in the animal's wool and can be used on any abused nipple of any age. Going *au natural* nips out has never been so invigorating! Fun for everyone!

Itchy nippies is no fun and uncovering the source of the aggravation can be tricky. Antihistamine tablets or creams have the ability to calm that intense itch. As always, when in doubt get that checked out by a healthcare professional. Treating the symptoms instead of the cause only delays the healing process. Any persistent concern could indicate a more serious illness so if you notice the nipple cream isn't improving the issue, don't wait too long to see a professional.

This advice is particularly important if discharge from the nipple is present. This brings us to the next segment where early detection can be a lifesaver.

Read My Nips: Cancer Screening

Bringing in the busty buoys for professional prevenative screenings can make all the difference in diagnosis and prognosis. Sure, it's not as fun or relaxing as the old Netflix and chill... But it is a necessary part of maintaining optimal levels of functionality to achieve a fulfilling life. Put down that remote, put on some clothes because you're going to the doctor. Prevention is key!

When the dreaded "c-word" creeps up into any conversation or consciousness, life screeches to a halt. Everything seems in slow motion and nothing else matters more than taking care of any nagging thoughts: What is this lump? What is this discharge? Why does my breast pucker like it had tasted a sour lemon? Why do my boobs hurt?

The amount of various questions could be endless but the answer is always: When in doubt, get it checked out.

Even having inverted nipples could be the result of an underlying malignancy or inflammatory illness. The sooner it is caught by healthcare professionals, the more options they may be able to present in treating the condition.

Cancer tends to have its own set of red flags, or markers. Asymmetrical areolas, distorted-looking nipples, and discharge are a few early warning signs that something isn't right. Monthly checks of the pecs can be as simple as holding your arm above your head while looking at the area in question in the mirror, searching for indentations or changes in the skin.

With your arm raised, massage the mammary tissue outward from the areola with your opposite hand. Follow this outward motion methodically around the entire breast area. Really feel yourself up! Repeat the process on the opposite side. The entire exam could be more fun with a partner. This also adds a second set of eyes, and hands, that may notice when something goes awry. The key takeaway here is to remain abreast of any changes to your body and get yourself evaluated by a healthcare professional if you have concerns.

Lumps, bumps, areas of the breast that feel hard or tender, unexplainable pain, or changes that seem out of the norm for you are all reasonable causes to get checked out. If you notice any of these in the underarm area, this could also indicate something amiss. Bring this up to your doctor at your next appointment, or sooner if it nags at the back of your mind like some gnat that you cannot be rid of no matter how you swat at it.

Speaking of things that nag and creep... Sometimes, age just creeps up on us and it is time to add more preventative screenings to our annual health checkups. Once a woman reaches age 50 or has cause for concern, the Centers for Disease Control and Prevention (CDC) recommends that mammograms become part of the routine checkup and images should be updated every two years. Being able to monitor changes in breast tissue over time means those mammaries will be fit to hang around that much longer. Any abnormality would be easily detected when comparing previous images to the most recent scans so keep up with those pesky appointments! They may pay off in the long run.

To evaluate your personal risk factors for developing breast cancer over your lifetime, it is imperative to consider family inheritance (the closer the relative, the higher the risk), sex (females inherently have a greater chance of getting breast cancer than males), and certain ethno-genetic factors that accompany people of color or those of Jewish heritige.

For example, Sauter, et al., conducted studies in 2002 to measure the similarities between, and note any ethnic differences in kallikrein, or the protein peptides that possess the power to direct physiological processes within the body. It gets a bit technical, but the end result is that researchers determined hK2 and hK3 levels in nipple aspiration fluid (NAF) remain low in black women in comparison to increased levels of these protein compounds found in white women. They also discovered a link between the presence of hK2 and hK3 in NAF and an elevated risk for breast cancer.

The same study also found that premenopausal levels of hK2 were lower in black females than in white females. This indicates that, in general, females who have yet to undergo "the change" known as menopause have a lower risk of developing breast cancer than women who have ceased the hormone secretions that regulate monthly menses. These findings also mean that white females in general are at an elevated risk for breast cancer when compared to the risk black females encounter for this same disease based on the level of these two peptides. However, this evaluation does not explain why, in reality when studying actual cases, black women are still at higher risk for developing breast cancer anyway or why they are more likely to succumb to the ravages of this disease.

One main difference in prognosis for these two demographics is that black women have a proportionately more difficlut time achieving adequate healthcare and are far more likely to put off or be refused for medical treatment due to lack of insurance coverage. So while breast cancer is more likely to happen to a white woman, she is better able to survive it. This disparity arises because societies make it so, not because the disease itself discriminates. In 2022, many people and global institutions are trying to change that to support more successful outcomes for all who are afflicted by this disease.

There is hope for a cure. There are several scientists and doctors diligently working around the clock to create new treatment options, early dectection technology, and ways to cure cancers of all kinds forever. This sounds reassuring, and it is to a point, but everyone regardless of skintone or sex should perform self-breast exams monthly to maintain a baseline comparison for future exams. Doctors aren't home with you to catch everything. You'll notice more quickly if something seems 'off' and be able to act that much quicker to get help if you take inventory of your own homeostasis, or daily level of feeling 'okay.' This is your baseline for comparison. Don't delay, examine yourself today!

Whether you are male, female, non-binary, transgender, agender, or are just a plain human being of any kind, please take care of yourself. Social stigma, fear, and anxiety be damned. Take a trusted support person with you so that you can relieve this stressful unknown and return to living the life you love and deserve.

To set your mind at ease, please get those elevated Mount Everests evaluated.

Chapter 5:

The Nipple Across Cultures

While it has been said—albeit by this book—no two northern mountain peaks are alike. And this is a good thing. Who wants to stare at the same Picasso forever? Unless you're married to it, I bet the answer is: not many. It should also be noted that within certain demographic populations, nipples do show certain similarities.

Family resemblances go beyond how cute grandma's nose looks on little Sally. Sometimes Petey just inherited his father's flathead screw-looking nipples and it can't be easily overlooked.

For instance, black people tend to be graced with supernumerary nipples more often than white people. Also within this population, inverted nipples are more common. Even among white populations, people of Italian inheritence tend to have more espresso-tone areolas. Genetic variability goes wild when it comes to pigmentation and who gets what genes to express which phenotype, these are the genetically encoded physical features that can be seen when looking at a living organism. It's complicated and not at all like painting where colors blend. There is a science to genetic inheritance.

Sometimes, nipple comparison goes beyond what can be seen with the naked eye. Cultural comparisons of such chest additions such as extra nipples and what they mean to different societies also play a role in rites of passage ceremonies, in selecting the right bride in arranged marriages, and in determining the purity of kinship relationships so that families retain their reputation. Witches marks, or large moles, on the body were seen as bad omens. Today, these may be diagnosed accurately as polythelia and the mole/nipple would be removed from the patient instead of the popular puritan pastime of burning someone alive. Let's never do that again. Communal bonfires are supposed to be fun.

When we move away from the Western world, we begin to realize that not everyone has the same opinion of a nipple. Let's put on a pair of existential glasses and view our surroundings from the fresh lens of someone who grew up in another culture, in another land far from wherever we call home.

Eastern Views of the Double-Peaked Mountains

Africa is a continent made from a mosaic of cultural richness. Here we will explain in further detail one example discussed earlier of how ethnic heritage can influence one's view of the appropriateness of nipple exposure in public and elsewhere. The Nigerian rite of passage ceremony that leads young women from "fattening rooms," where they are pampered sampling decadent foods and enjoying luxuries like watching television and being fanned by family members as relief from unbearably hot temperatures, through purity examinations and finally into the realm of marriage can be grueling (Onwurah and Gardner, 1993). Customs such as these may seem barbaric to outsiders.

The value this tradition has for these people cannot be measured by today's standards or by Western worldviews. In the ethnographic film *Monday's Girls*, film creators Onwurah and Gardner (1993) follow three young Nigerian women as they prepare to take part in this coming-of-age ceremony that will be viewed by the entire village and overseen by respected elders. There were young nugs on display and no one objected even if they did objectify by Western standards of moral conduct. There is no guarantee that the exposed females were over 18 which is considered the age of majority in most countries.

This differs greatly from the Western consternation of averting everyone's eyes from even a gentle nip-slip. Nudity is a no-no!

As the group of initiates was paraded through the village, topless and exposed but generally proud to participate, there truly were no visible signs one could use to determine the girls' purity, which was the point of the entire shebang! A bride-to-be is more desirable as a virgin than if she has been plucked, supposedly. Here's one instance where years of experience apparently gets you nowhere. Don't tell that to your potential employer! The two topics are not mutually exclusive and it may be considered bad manners to even bring it up. You've been jovially warned.

Everyone was searching for evidence of darkened areolas and engorged breasts that would indicate prior pregnancy (and therefore sexual impurity) in this culture. But the village elders (all male) smiled and stared. Reading these nipples was a matter of embracing the responsibilities placed upon everyone by their inherited way of life. Everyone had a role to play. That's just always how it had been for them.

One culture may claim this is wrong while another may be in full support like the pushiest push-up bra this side of Victoria's Secret.

The point is that the world exists as a wild thing. Wild things grow against their own set of rules and no other set of rules could truly apply universally. After all, every vine seeks sunshine. Some vines just have more thorns or need less water than others. It simply is.

Industrialized Ice Caps

Modern modesty is nothing new, and it certainly isn't simple. Before the Industrial Revolution began around 1793 in the U.S., there were women labeled schoolmarms or tramps. Women were either "frigid" or "hot to trot." There was very little left to label in between. And label everything they did!

Reclaiming words that used to bear negative connotations like 'bitch' and 'slut' have proved empowering for some. Even to the extent that pop songs grew edgier in the '90s with Meredith Brooks's hit 'Bitch,' subversive titles meant to demean women if they dare bare their cleavage or their teeth have been turned into anthems for rebellion.

Meredith Brooks belted out lyrics like (1997):

> Yesterday I cried, you must have been relieved to see the softer side. I can understand how you'd be so confused; I don't envy you. I'm a little bit of everything all rolled into one: I'm a bitch, I'm a lover, I'm a child, I'm a mother. I'm a sinner, I'm a saint. I do not feel ashamed. I'm your hell; I'm your dream. I'm nothing in between. You know you wouldn't want it any other way. So take me as I am.

Here we get an eyeful, or an earful rather. Who doesn't love a bad girl? Would we want her or anyone any other way?

No, history has been clear that rebellious women make history. Sitting down nips all demure doesn't get the job done (generally speaking). So how does the mainstream media explain the complicated relationship between someone being an acceptable tramp and someone who is tormented for daring to be authentically trailblazing? The answer remains unknown. It's a fine line to walk for sure but these boots were made for walking after all.

Rebels: We love to hate them.

And the media play both sides. They can twist a titty shot as artistic or vulgar. Even across different eras, the story is the same: the duality of female sexuality is always under scrutiny. Certainly, someone at the time thought Rosie the Riveter was hot and got the hots for the triangular titillations beneath her denim jumpsuit as she helped win World War II. Torpedoes away! But no one was policing the makers of these 'udderly' uncomfortable brassieres that gave women in the 1940s such unnaturally shaped breasts.

Bullet bras became the accepted form of underwear to demurely cover women's breasts (lifting breast tissue away from the chest that encased the areolas into incredibly sharp, perpendicular points) during the 1940s. For twenty years after, it was worn by women nationwide in the U.S. and elsewhere, bolstered by the war effort and later reinforced as the epitome of femininity by the newly invented and exclusively viewed home television set. These uncomfortable torture devices disguised as proper female attire were created as a way to shape the female body in a subtly alluring way while also adhering to the strict modesty standards set by people unofficially dubbed the "prude police."

Sex symbols on the silver screen like blonde bombshell Marilyn Monroe donned these bullet bras as they embraced the snug satin and lace restrictions of their time. Society expected them to conform to this form-fitting attire while simultaneously displaying a coy demeanor. Fully dressed in satin and sex, icons like Monroe pushed back against this bipolar love-hate battle of the boobs and were still demonized for their vapid vulgarness even when every naughty bit was covered.

Marilyn Monroe's assignment as a starlet-harlot probably stemmed from her breathy voice, the vivacious and graceful way she moved her body across the motion picture screen, and the way her hooded eyes beckoned the audience to join her in the bedroom. None of this supposedly sinful 'sex' was overt, everything was implied or exaggerated beyond its original intent.

These subtleties in how others interpret someone's existence as 'female' still haunts women, girls, and transwomen alike. Unrealistic and unfair assessments rear their ugly, misogynistic heads in policies like school dress codes that target spaghetti straps and skirt lengths while omitting any such restrictions on the male appearance. The theory goes that *no one* wants to see someone else's nipples but it sure seems like it really all stems from *everyone* wanting to know what goes on beneath a person's clothing.

This wouldn't be a problem if society went by prehistoric principles: Everyone was naked and no one cared. Nipples pre-date human existence and yet their acceptance into the public eye is shaped by a supposedly intellectual, moral public opinion so much so that they get a bad rap. We honestly cannot blame the nipples here, just the boobs.

Western Whoas vs. Woes

Western culture is considered to include North America (the United States of America and Canada), the UK, most European countries, Australia, Norway, Iceland, and New Zealand. This is because the socio-economic situations and customs present in each place have relatively similar characteristics: These include comparable governments like democracy, having an individualistic viewpoint rather than a collectivistic one, using similar technological systems and devices, and possessing similar religious beliefs (most dominantly being Christianity).

As boring as a history lesson right now might be, we're here to educate. Sometimes the only way forward is to examine where we originated. Early in its inception, Europe loved to explore and conquer things, animals, people, and places. While we know this is wrong and harmful today, the world that existed way back when viewed everything a bit differently.

When we know better, we do better.

Wherever Europeans traveled they shared their religious and cultural beliefs while egregiously erasing large portions of the cultures and people they wanted to homogenize. Sharing, shearing… The end result was the same. Everywhere they went, European ways of life became the new normal in several countries where already established values had been the norm since time immemorial.

Modesty culture is a result of austere religious expectations and thus is born a majority of anti-nipple nuns in the habit of hiding their conical coifs in exchange for a promised afterlife.

We're here to party now! So while tribal cultures were forced to cover their chests and confine their carnal coins, recent activists who call for equality are bringing the nipple back into the spotlight for sunlight to shed light on what needs to be done to rectify such an imbalance of human rights. For starters: Free the nipple!

Bare breasts are permitted on certain nude beaches and are acceptable (protected from a legal standpoint) in specific situations such as while breastfeeding. But there has been tremendous pushback in recent years, as is evidenced by social media campaigns like #FreetheNipple and slogans like My Body, My Choice.

Being able to bare both soul and breast the same as any male is incredibly liberating and validating for every human being but always be mindful of safety. When in foreign countries with their own laws and ideas of morality, knowing your local limitations may mean the difference between a successful, happy vacation and being arrested.

At least on the homefront, keep up the good fight, nips ablazing, because not every country permits its citizens to disagree so publicly with its policies no matter how respectfully the outcry is orchestrated.

Chapter 6:

Modesty! Politics! Nipples!

There isn't much left in life that isn't considered political. "Go woke, go broke" is the new mantra for the masses. Sure, it's catchy and it rhymes. Years ago, there were certain topics that just were not discussed due to their potential to start an argument at the dinner table. These were traditionally topics of religious, political, or financial regard. Really, who wants indigestion while eating what should have been a peaceful, delicious family meal?

But sometimes, silence is compliance and basic human rights should not be up for debate. The end result seems to be families divided and turbulent pockets of people nationwide willing to argue with strangers at the drop of a hat. The internet is full of social media Jerry Springer-style virtual brawls so audiences grab a bucket of popcorn and get their fill of the verbal violence that regrettably can lead to actual physical violence.

And here we are talking about nipples.

Nipples are natural. Breasts are functional. But the problem is that breasts can be fun, too.

Hiding the nipple is like taking away a child's favorite toy that lights up. This is primarily why those cherry tarts are policed so hard: They could create tantrums and bad behavior from those who view them. These covetous cones are a sight to behold, and those who spy them may want to hold them, so the solution has been to cover the areolas to take away the temptation.

Sure, it's not fair to place blame on the jewelry store for displaying such glittering baubles when it is the thief who crossed the line and tarnished the tinsel.

Beauty is the eye of the beholder so should the blame also lie. What a wonderful world it would be if anyone who wanted to bare their beautiful bosom never had to spare a passing thought to self-safety or worry about being arrested or accosted. Blessed be the boob.

Being Prudish

Intriguing and illegal: breast meats of any kind in the human form have been banned, beguiled, and wrongfully blamed for all manner of wrong-doing mostly perpetrated by men who don't even own these bouncy balloons. Men are everywhere. We're making the laws. We're enforcing the laws. But dammit we want to see these things, so why are we making it so hard on ourselves?

The simple answer is that most of us have wives and daughters. Our wives would rather we only lust after their busts and as for our daughters, we don't want to believe they even have breasts.

It's the belief that boobies are out there, there are ones we haven't seen, that fuels our curiosity. There are ones we could only ever dream of seeing. So many mysteries surround the neverending need to view, to hold, or to motorboat the bobbing buoys of our fantasies. There exist a plethora of possibilities that every combination of breast tissue, skin tone, areola size and shape, innie, outie, wonky, oddly-shaped, mismatched and attributes yet to be discovered could be right there. And we just have to know!

Humans are blessed and cursed by their curiosity.

Being able to explore the natural world is no exception. One of nature's blessings has been the existence of the breast and we just want to be able to steal a glance if one graces our sightlines. The reason we are mostly unable to do so is because of consequences.

Like the dog who caught up to the tire after giving chase for two solid blocks, we'd be rolled for miles once we got home. Wives are lovely but they are not very understanding when it comes to explaining away how we risked one eye to peep at someone's peaks as they picked up whatever they dropped.

And just like that, we're sleeping in the doghouse. And that's only *if* we survive the initial grilling. So the solution has become to keep the temptations to a minimum by passing laws, enforcing those laws, and keeping the peace for more than the public. We have to keep the peace at home too if we ever hope to have a piece of the piece we married before bed each night.

Policing the Areola

We've already covered #FreetheNipple (haha), so let's introduce you to another expression of body equality: #Topfreedom. Consider this the sister set willing to bat for the right to dress up or dress down any nipple regardless of whatever sex, age, or level of sexiness the nipple owner embodies as long as they're of legal and consenting age.

While the jury is still out on the legitimacy of the Topfree Equality Rights Association (TERA) situated in Canada that claims to help any female facing legal repercussions for freeing their chest jubblies, it seems as though many places outside of North America are more relaxed regarding releasing the chest raisins in public.

Breast tissue, side boob, under-boob, every boob, entire boob, impotent boobs and dumb nipples… What makes the areola so criminal?

The issue seems to be that it is illegal for women to turn men on with their booby bullseyes. When *Men's Health* ran an article in 2015 asking this very question, criminal defense attorney Jeffrey J. Douglas, who practices in Santa Monica, California, was interviewed and that was his answer.

Here again, the responsibility for the boner is placed in women's hands and not in the lap of the man who owns the wood. Being held accountable is hard. We can do better.

What could humankind accomplish if it wasn't always plagued by being so prudish? Thinking like a stuffy, curmudgeony chaperone for the chaste 24/7 instead of being a coquettish, flirty and fun-loving filly only serves as a disservice to everyone everywhere. Bottled animosity leads to unhealthy ways of expressing that natural, animalistic side of being human. Embracing our inner carefree, frisky foal seems like a much healthier way of life than worrying constantly over the amount of cleavage in existence. Other animals don't worry about others seeing their udders and teats. If we're being honest, cleavage is the least of the world's worries and absolutely no one is shoving it in other people's faces. I know. I've looked. I was just as disappointed as you are.

But! One ray of areolar sunshine remains unexplored: Nude nipple lipstick! It's flirty, it conveys a kind of friskiness, and it mimics nature. *But how do I pick a color that will compliment my face?*, you may ask. It's all about matching the drapes to the carpet… well, kind of.

One of the oddest things about having areolas is that there is so much that is genuinely natural about them, it's practically a crime to keep them under such harsh scrutiny. We've never pushed so hard to free the nipple as now because this is a matter of fashion!

Take natural lip color for example. Did you know that the best way to choose a natural, true-to-you shade is by first knowing what color your areolas are? We're talking more than just a smart cherry chapstick. So how in the world would anyone ever even guess what color that is with all that fabric in the way? We don't know and it's a good question.

Dusty rose bust bipples? There's a lipstick to match that! Are your areolas more merlot? Revlon has a rainbow of hues to mimic whatever nipple you were blessed to bestow. Now the whole world can know, too, without ever *truly* knowing. You know?

Using your nipples like dowsing rods to locate the correct nude lip shade may not always work. One reason is that nipple color is influenced by hormonal changes. Nips get darker during pregnancy or with sun exposure. Younger areolas are usually lighter in hue which might end up washing out your facial features if you match lipstick to nipply-bits. Try before you buy but do yourself a favor and check the color of your nips at home, take a selfie, keep it secret, keep it safe…rather than busting that bust out and comparing L'Oréal to the real thing at the cosmetics counter. Macy's will thank you.

Don't even get us started on the newest trend of matching your face-lips to the shade of your naughty nightshade ladybits. It's already gotten weird enough and there's a lot of pink involved.

Desexualizing, unfetishizing parts of the female body like picking the choicest cuts of meat at the butcher's block is the best place to begin in defunding the areola police. When the nipple is locked away beneath bras and shirts, coats, and clothing in general instead of being brought out to enjoy the sun like an everyday nipple, the thrill becomes less shocking a sight. Desensitize what thoughts arise inside the onlooker and decriminalize the milk duds. The less sexually the world views breasts, the happier the breast bearers will become. Everyone else will benefit, too.

This way we can all one day hold up in hearty comparison our boob-tubes to lipstick tubes in hopes of finding the *perfect* nip-lip color for us!

It would be so much easier, and honestly more fun, to be topfree in public while shopping and eating in restaurants. No more unnecessary mess by spilling spaghetti on our shirts! Stains would become virtually nonexistent! That sounds like a win-win for everyone. Keep the kibble away from the kebabs…you don't want torched titties! We're always trying to keep you abreast of any foreseeable dangers. You're welcome.

Breast is ALWAYS Best

Nope, this is not another breastfeeding anthem! We've covered the topic as thoroughly as anyone possibly could without outright shoving it too far down anyone's throat. Breastfed babies have it nice… But that's not the point of this section.

Wherever there are breasts, there is surely also someone somewhere close nearby who is in want of breasts. A budding child praying to the titty gods for a c-cup, *Grow little boobies grow, grow, grow.* Sometimes we've even heard our little sisters utter such prayers for udders while they attempted uncomfortable exercises aimed at enlarging the areas in question. Poor child, that is unfortunately not how it works. Pull a tissue from your stuffed booby-trap and wipe your eyes. You'll grow into it one day. There is no rush so enjoy the freedom of youth as long as you can. It's all downhill after the peak.

On the flipside, there are several other adults who long to be held near and dear to a perky pair of gargantuan globules or grab some gonzagas as they search the earth for their soulmate… or regular mate. Doing it like they do on the Discovery Channel…

Just because someone owns a pair of breasts does not imply they have to commit to doing anything they deem uncomfortable with those bouncy buoys. Ownership does not imply consent for unwanted touching or looking or leering or cheering. Display cases were not meant to be open to the public for groping. Someone fine and sexy needs no applause, they know they're hot so let them trot in peace! We look with our eyes, not with our hands. That'd be weird.

Booby does not imply duty. Ogling or brushing a breast is an unwanted assault.

Anything less than an emphatic YES means no. And this applies to any point even if consent was originally given, it can be revoked at any point. So play nice.

When you finally are welcomed into that high-vibration, double-heaping helping of honey-dough goodness, be grateful. Motorboating between two breasts is where so many people wish they could be and will sadly never attain.

Chapter 7

Free the Nipple!

The nip outcry heard 'round the world, via Instagram and Facebook, of course; Free the nipple! This campaign gained traction around 2019, with the hashtag donning over 4 million posts. Even in photos of cancer survivors where all nipples have been surgically removed via mastectomy, Instagram still takes offense and takes these posts down.

According to the superficial explanation by the companies' representatives, they are merely "keeping within the bounds of social propriety: If you walked down the street in New York, one employee explained, you wouldn't see exposed female nipples on advertisements" (Jacobs, 2019). Hogwash!

Did you know that in NYC any person can walk around topless regardless of how much mammary meat they are packing? It's true! Since 1992, being bare-chested anywhere in New York state has been completely legal (Peralta, 2015). Specifically, anywhere a man can be topless, so can a woman be as long as no one is paying for the view. Thus making Instagram's overly prudish statement completely null.

For the record, we're all in for what is good for the goose being also good for the gander. Who doesn't like to gander from time to time?

Feminism Can Be Feminist

Showing skin in consensual, performative ways for the greater good is an incredibly noble cause. As mentioned above, the 1992 ruling on the New York State penal code 245.01 previously stated that revealing "private or intimate parts of one's body" was punishable by law, singling out the female body specifically to incldue showing breast tissue "which is below the top of the areola" in public (Peralta, 2015). What is a crime for women is just fine for men.

Needless to say, members of society who felt singled out weren't going to take it anymore. The 1992 ruling began in 1986 with two women who decided their goose was as good as any man's gander. Summer solstice 1986 arrives and Ramona Santorelli and Mary Lou Schloss were two of nine women who would execute their staged, very public, topfree picnic in the park to prove a point. Of course, they are arrested for lewd misconduct and charged with indecent exposure.

These fearless females fought back. The Fourteenth Amendment guaranteed that they were to be treated as equals to men. This should include how they are able to present their bodies in public. If men are able to go nips out, surely females (having nipples also) should be free to do the same. No one ever criticizes their crusty nubs or arrests them for baring their beastly breasts, after all.

Dropping the criminal charges was not enough. These women wanted equality. Ramona Santorelli and Mary Lou Schloss continued their court battle on behalf of womenkind everywhere and they won! Nipple equality was achieved in New York!

By standing their ground and pursuing the initial issue, Schloss and Santorelli were able to create a more feminist interpretation of New York state law. Feminism means equality between all people. Any future court cases of this nature that call into question the presence of discrimination would need to refer back to this ruling as a guide. It helped to set a precedent for other state's laws and progressed human rights to a more equitable condition.

Feminism is not a dirty word. It doesn't mean that women should rule and men should drool. To clear up any uncertainty about what feminism is, it is *not* the opposite of chauvinism or patriarchy. Both of the latter thrive through subjugating several specific minorities such as people of color, impoverished individuals, differently-abled people, and female or other gender-identifying groups excluding cisgender white males.

Cisgender individuals identify as the sex they were assigned at birth. Don't let these terms ruffle your feather and PLEASE refrain from ripping this book to shreds! See…just about anything can be perceived as political. Terms like 'feminism' and 'cisgender' originated in sociology through the study of societies. This doesn't automatically make them dirty words or political at all.

There is no agenda here, only the humble offering of information. Nipple information is pertinent for everyone because most people are born with their own set! That's real equality!

The point is that true feminism is when each person within their own body gains every control to show or conceal as little or as much as they wish of themselves as they lead the life they are free choose. Body autonomy and ability to live a life unfettered should be the floor, not the ceiling.

A Modern Movement Making Waves

Hashtag Free the Nipple has been a cause for many years before it began trending on social media sites like Facebook and Instagram. It began in the United States in the face of social media censorship that applied to women (only) who were openly breastfeeding, women who'd undergone mastectomies to combat breast cancer, females in art and photography, and as a war cry in general at the inequality of having their areolas "silenced" because of misogynistic modesty regulations. Misogyny is defined as outright prejudice against females and the world is rife with it.

Have you ever heard that it's a man's world? This is due mostly to the fact that men are elected to and hold the highest government offices. They make the rules most places where women exist. So while women have been hitting their heads against a glass ceiling of prejudice and discouragement in every building (or socio-political realm) they occupy (guess who insallted that glass ceiling? Yep, that was us, too) most recently that has begun to change. Images of breastfeeding were just accepted by social media giants as late as 2014 due to the persistent protests and awareness raised by human rights activists who refuse to stay silent anymore (Jacobs, 2019).

But there's more to women than their nipples or what they could offer someone sexually.

The January 2017 Women's March across the U.S. was a smash hit that helped everyone realize this. Knowing that the president-elect of 2016 would attempt to chip away at all the social progress Americans had fought to be made, 5 million women, allies, and other supporters took to big-city streets to conduct the largest congregation of activists in the history of the world.

With pink pussy hats complete with kitty cat-shaped ears ('pussy' get it?) atop their heads and protest signs at the ready, women gathered in riotous uproar to exercise their First Amendment right to free speech and to assemble peacefully. Their voices were heard loud and clear despite there being not much else that could be done to remedy the impending Jenga-style removal of common sense laws that would span several areas of concern, failing to renew the repercussions guaranteed to deter anyone from violating the Violence Against Women Act, or further restricting the reproductive and healthcare decisions a female could make.

Make no mistake: When legal precedents have been set and social progress that promotes equality among humankind alike is passed into law, everyone in society should move forward to tackle the next big problem rather than revert to beating dead horses over and over again. It's dead, it's buried. Let's leave it to see what grows from the fresh dirt.

We march forward together, or we march leaving some behind running to catch up…It is hoped that we're all in it together as a collective humankind.

Undressing Modesty Culture

Men can bare their breasts, even those that are larger than some female cup sizes. So what makes a female nipple different from a male nipple in the eyes of the public?

It has been argued that one reason for the exclusive censorship of the female areola is due to it being considered an erogenous zone, comparatively covered by the same public guidelines set for genital exposure. It is universally considered lewd and criminal to flash what you've got going on below the belt anywhere within public view.

Erroneously, the individuals who make the rules have deemed a nipple unsexy only if it belongs to a man. But this is more a comment on personal perception rather than a fact that male nipples aren't erogenous zones for male pleasure. In all actuality, that is the only purpose of male nipples: being useful for sexual stimulation.

As discussed earlier in the anatomy of male and female nippies, it has been revealed that the majority of nipples have numerous nerves that cause them to be sensitive. So yes, nipples can be useful in sexual arousal for both men and women. So the argument then becomes that the only difference between the female nipple and its male counterpart is that when the nipple belongs to a woman, it magically possesses the ability to sexually arouse the person peering at it. Are men not afforded the same level of attractiveness? How rude to assume!

Therefore, the message sent by social media, mass media, and public policy, in general, is that because females *could* be seen as sexy, they *must* cover themselves or risk inciting a genital inferno that the viewer may not be able to control. We're calling bull! The only person in control of one's own actions is oneself. There's no one else to blame.

Placing this kind of control on the female body rather than on the voyeur sends a dangerous and absolutely discriminatory message to women everywhere: Cover up or face the consequences however criminal they may be.

What was she wearing? *She had it coming*, might be overhead if the victim comes forward to press charges. This unjust shaming and unsupportive aftercare in place for any victimized person is known as rape culture which only propogates placing blame back on the victim instead of punishing the predator. Surely the people writing the rules find it easier to censor ownership of the boobs than to hold accountable the people who wish to act on the boobs. This doesn't make it right. This is why we march. No one hears nice girls when they ask politely, nipples all demure. We should stand in solidarity with our bosom companions to make their lives a bit easier.

Yet another injustice: The theory in play also appears to be that the same people who are part of the nipple police get all the fun. They view the supposed lewdness (win) and then bear no consequences for their lecherous thoughts and most of the time their actions on those thoughts while placing the blame for the situation on the nipple bearer (also win). All play and no penalties. Score for them! Boo for everyone else.

But the truth is evident. And this misogynistic mammary-minding needs to be revised so that all nipples are equal. Free the nipple! And the rest will follow.

Chapter 8:

Know Thy Nipple, Know Thyself!

Customer complaints are high these days. A plethora of people on this planet means fewer resources, less arm room on airplanes, and longer lines at Disney World. Yeah, we see you!

But while people genuinely necessitate the world going on along some semblance of normal, we know life can ultimately get you down.

It's been said that customers are always right. Whatever makes the customer happy, make the pocket change rain! This seems like the case for everyone regardless of nipple condition. That being said, while it's raining nips for some there are also those who are experiencing a nip-drip drought and are none too happy about it.

Feeling less than stellar about your self-image has the diabolical ability to make people desperate. This can manifest as countless plastic surgeries, diet fads for weight loss, and buying more costumes to disguise our unhappiness than could be found in all the dressing rooms of Las Vegas. Speaking of Las Vegas, pack your bags and bring clean socks because we're going there soon by way of breast augmentation! So grab your beach gear, we're going to be talking mammoth flotation devices soon!

Let's explore a few ways nips dictate the ways humans behave.

What If I Have No Nips?

This condition would be known as athelia and it is incredibly rare. You should play the lottery with those odds. Although it is likely inherited, athelia is usually a result of other medical conditions such as Poland's.

Autosomal dominant inheritance be damned, you can still have your nips and dress them, too! Who's going to tell you how to live your life: no one!

Nipple transplants could be in your future. Just know that the research and results are still experimental at the time of this writing.

Other options could be going under the needle instead of the knife. I hear they're doing lovely things with nipples at your local tattoo shop these days. Find yourself a reputable, talented tatter to tat those tits. It is painful, but if you've got the dedication and money it may just be worth your while.

One last-ditch effort is to accept who you are in all your glory, no nips and all. You are wonderful just the way you are. It's like I tell my kids, if someone has a problem with you for something you have no control over, then they aren't very good 'friends' anyway. You can do better!

Treat yourself like a king, queen, marsupial…whatever makes you happy. But you've got to be able to live with yourself at the end of the day; at the end of every day, really. Live and let live!

I Am More Than My Pair of Headlights

To reinforce this fierce philosophy of living and letting live, we make our way to discussing the art of decadently dancing the nipple from its home in a glittering, provacative halter top for profit. Yep, you guessed it! We're talking exoctic dancers twirling tassels in ways we never thought possible. Their graceful efforts should be rewarded generously. Dancing at a skeevy titty bar might make the bills, but does it heighten your sense of self-worth? If you answered 'yes' we commend your sassy spirit!

No one should feel ashamed for how they choose to bolster their bustier in hopes of making money. After all, in the U.S. and around the world, labor economies built by our bodies is what makes the big bucks for our employers. Wages are exchanged for time and wear and tear on our minds and bodies is the same as it would be if we dressed up to dance for tips.

While some may decide to look down upon these dancers in the dark, understand that they're making a living. They're people, too. They have nipples and bills and feelings, hopes and dreams the same as most anyone else.

If you're someone who is looking down from that flashy pole, know that we're here to spill the beans about your pasties.

That's right: These adhesives come in all shapes, colors, patterns, and sizes. The best part is they are sometimes reusable so they don't have to be thrown away immediately.

These and titty tape are sometimes used by celebrities during award shows or during intimate scenes on the big screen. Those nip slips can be costly! Recall the early discussion about Nipplegate 2004.

Like their more decorative sisters, the titty tassel sticks onto the flesh encompassing the areola. There's just a bit more to this ornament than a lick-em stick-em adhesive. Dangling down from the center of the provocative pasty is a colorful stream of entwined strings. These entrance the eye as the tassels sway with every minute motion the wearers make. Twirling faster one side, and slower on the other or making them move in unison, clockwise, counterclockwise, and even some acrobatic arrays not many have had the pleasure of viewing.

Whether you're playing with the tassels meant to adorn curtains as you walk the aisles of Hobby Lobby, or you're a pro that makes the tassels go, know that we know your trade secrets. Knowing makes us no less curious so we'll still be watching you… In a non-stalker way of course. Like we've mentioned before, humans are a curious bunch.

You may ask how anyone could get away with only covering the bare necessities. After all, if the majority of the breast is visible then doesn't it stand to reason that the *whole* thing is still lascivious? The long and short of it is, no. There are exceptions made for all other areas of the breast to be shown, even underboob, the only exclusion is the female areola. That's a no-no. In rare cases, even the subtle shadow of deepening rose or cacao can be spied trying to overstep the line of permissibility and these moments are permitted onscreen as acceptable. Just don't hit the bullseye and you'll be fine. The outskirts of the nipple area barely squeak through modesty filters but make a way, they often do.

How does society both lust after and shun breasts, specifically the nipple? There's a long line of psychological, theological, and patriarchal undertones fueling this conundrum.

Suffice it to say that somewhere along the way, someone got their knickers in a twist over an exposed breast and ruined the whole experience for everyone. What a party pooper.

Understanding What Your Nipples Are Saying

It may be too hot in here, and we may want to take off all our clothes but societal norms have dictated we remain clothed. So we sweat.

Understanding the art of nipple reading is no easy task. Best to mind your own mammaries on this one. Knowing when to fan the fleshy chest-fritters and when to pile on the layers can be a bit complicated.

When hormone levels become erratic this can cause sweating, where the body, the hands, and face become flushed with 'boiling' blood. We pull at the collars of our shirts and fan our hands in front of our faces like we're on fire to no avail.

Inadvertently, our nipples and underarms begin to secrete salty sweat that sometimes stinks!

So we pull at our clothing even more hoping that this small gust of cool air finds its way down the neck-hole of our favorite button-up. This doesn't work either. It seems like nothing is appeasing the mammary gland gods so we make lame excuses to excuse ourselves… My cat's calling me or I left the coffee pot on (even at 11 o'clock at night!). How embarrassing.

These social *faux pas* may haunt us for the rest of our lives, but not as deeply as if we'd sweated right through our shirts.

How do nipples even leak sweat? We've learned that they sometimes leak milk from a lactating person's breasts. Even males may experience leakage from draining lymphatic liquid. But sweat is another story.

Nipples are porous in more than just their blind lactiferous ducts or their deep channels of functional lactiferous sinuses. Pores appear as microscopic openings along the skin's surface. Sometimes these orifices become clogged and pimples, blackheads, or whiteheads appear. The presence of pores equates to the presence of sweat glands (sweat, dirt, and bacteria all build blockages and lead to breakouts).

Remember the Montgomery tubercles? Yep, those bumps around the areola are indeed sweat glands. They can become clogged so it is best to wash yourself following an intense workout… or other cardio-intensive activities (wink wink).

When hot, boobs sweat. When frigid temperatures have your nips shaking in their shirts, it's time to break out the lightweight layers (preferably cotton because it 'breathes') and keep those chilly ice caps cloaked in mystery.

Choosing the right fabric, natural over synthetic, will increase the health and happiness of the two most hyper-critical hecklers your chest will ever carry. Keeping the nips covered in layers means they won't be likely to interrupt your flirtations at the company Christmas party because some chilly wind catches your nip *en guard*!

Likewise, if you are worried about letting down while in the nursing stage of your baby's early development, you can skip the breastmilk nip-slip-n-slide by wearing absorbent breast pads inside your bra. They may be a pain to hold onto while your infant is actively nursing. One fun suggestion is to place the circular, somewhat conical fabric circle on the back of your child's head: instant *yamaka*! Breast Pads are useful and fun! Consider them to be a party hat for your party hats.

Machine washable, cotton breast pads are safe for daily use. The alternative is synthetic, plastic-feeling disposable breast pads and since honesty is the best policy: You should know that wearing disposable booby blotters feels just about as comfortable as wearing plastic panty liners all day in the blistering sun. Or so I've been told because, gratefully-speaking, I've never worn either of them. It sounds like slip 'n' slide city with none of the fun. You may feel sweaty and gross so it's recommended to use the cotton ones that are machine washable. You're welcome in advance.

So do everyone, but especially yourself, a favor: Read your nips, and often!

Breast Augmentation, or Rearranging the Nips

If you've ever been to Las Vegas… You've surely seen a pair (or several pairs) of augmented breasts. They draw the eye to the chest because our subconscious is pondering how such perky boobs could exist in the natural world. The truth is, it took surgical magic and a lot of recovery time, painkillers, and a small fortune to create those covetous cones. While they may not feel like natural breasts in they way they mold to the shape of your hand, implants do have their perks.

One advantage to getting a boob job is that the recipient doesn't really require the support of a bra any longer. Those two pert sisters hold up nicely all on their own. This saves so much money in the lingerie department and is vastly more comfortable than squeezing into a push-up bra where the tops of your twin peaks meets your chin. No one wants to be strangled by their skin mountains.

There are a couple options available to fill in your sandbags. Synthetic breast implants are made of silicone or saline. These can decompose over time, so once the skin is stretched out, these implants will need to be replaced every few decades in order to maintain the desired shape and aesthetic of a larger breast.

Cup sizes vary! If you've ever wanted to supersize anything, here's your chance. Cup size changes depending on the amount of fluid injected into the insert: Know that anything over 400cc is considered large and the smallest size available is 150cc. Even within the two types of implants there are three shapes from which to choose. The textured teardrop, the textured round, and the smooth round are all viable options.

If the desired effect is a full bosom, round is your best breast... I mean bet. The smooth variety is more comparable to the feel of touching a natural breast. Supposedly this is true, I wouldn't personally know but this is what I've been told so don't tell my wife. Hers are spectacular and are the only pair for me.

Others are not as satisfied with their juggernauts. Sagging breasts prior to the procedure, otherwise known as ptosis, would require a breast lift in addition to the surgical placement of a breast implant for the procedure to be successful. A boob job without a chesty facelift is doomed to fail with torpedoes pointed away from their target. A bad boob job is worse than no boob job. Please explore all pros and cons, side effects and possible long-term complications of altering what nature gave you because once its gone, there's no getting it back.

A patient could even personalize which profile they find most appealing and go for that implant shape. Choices for this category include the mini, demi, full, or ultra-high profile breast. As you can imagine, the last kind offers the more dramatic projection away from the chest wall. By default, these are also going to be the heaviest so choose wisely. Talk about a built in bullet bra because that's what this choice would look like. Anchors away!

Luckily, before the first cut, there are a few meetings with the surgeon to determine which size, shape, kind, and profile best fits the frame you'll be dressing with your new knockers. Computer programs are able to modify a photo of your body as is and then make the suggested alterations as a way to give you a realistic look at the results for what you can expect to achieve with surgery. Plastic surgeons are not magicians. And honestly, you're beautiful the way you are. We do understand if there are still changes you'd feel more comfortable making and we're not here to make them for you.

So have fun and do your thing!

This book is about nipples after all, so I'd be remiss if I missed the opportunity to tell you about how nipples are affected by getting breast implants. First, breastfeeding no longer becomes an option. Mammary glands, lobules, and lactiferous sinues become blocked or interrupted and all of a sudden a playground is built where a nursery had been. There are exceptions to every rule so be sure to check with your physician before surgery if you wish to breastfeed in the future.

Secondly, it is important to understand how nipple sensation may be affected in their rearrangement during surgery. As the breast tissue is pulled away from the pectoralis major muscle, nerve damage is likely to occur. This means less innervation, and possibly fewer nipple stimulated orgasms in your future. What a bummer.

Nipples, even on a good day, can get all cock-eyed and point in opposite directions. These compass needles may need redirection correction after a less-than-satisfactory breast augmentation so be forewarned. Breast tissue, adhesions, and scar tissues build up over time and may also cause nipples to migrate from where they were placed during surgery.

When dropping between $6,000 and $15,000 on such a prominent part of yourself in making a memorable first impression, you expect everything to be done right. Unfortunately, sometimes you get what you pay for and even that does not guarantee a lifetime of painfree play time with your repurposed dirty (now clean) pillows.

The surgery itself is outpatient with a recovery time of roughly one week. Let your body guide your tolerance level as you ease into regular daily activities after that. If everything goes to plan, and you're thrilled with your conical commitment: We're equally elated for you!

After all, a person who is pleased with their appearance is generally happier and more successful. More power to you! But so you know, we like you any way you are.

Chapter 9:

Learning to Love Your Nips

There are many, and I mean *many*, ways a person can love their nipples. Choosing fancy silver jewels to dangle from these precious peaks, engaging in an invigorating exfoliating nipple scrub, and even just giving the twins a soothing massage every so often are excellent ways to show your chesticles that you care. After all, they are the only set of nipples you will (probably) ever own. This makes them irreplaceable… Unless, of course, you desire to get a replacement set tattooed over what had been your original set if you ever have them removed for whatever reason. For everyone's sake, we hope you don't.

The point is that your nipples are yours, and yours alone. They will never belong to anyone else. This is the sheer beauty of being a nipple owner. No one else can tell you how best to wear your brazen booby buttons. So show them off in some sheer, gossamer garments all you like!

Self-Love

Oh nipples, how do I love you… Let me count the ways. Better yet: Let's take a moment to pause in all this nipple knowledge and appreciate the chest or breast for its truly amazing existence. Regardless of how you may feel about your own nipples, their size, their color, their peach fuzz, their absence, or any other characteristic, you can rest assured knowing that your nipples are nature's way of dressing up your own existence.

Whatever they look like, nipples help make you unique. So take care of your nips. Follow along to learn how.

Special care and cleansing of the nipples requires only clean, warm water. Astringents like soap can cause irritation, dryness, and can interfere with the body's ability to produce natural oil from the areolar glands.

For breastfeeding moms, moisture can be replenished to the nipple by expressing a bit of breastmilk and gently rubbing it into the areola area. Lanolin ointment, or natural oil found in lamb wool, can also be applied to the nipple if it is damaged or sore from a poor latch during nursing. Applying warm compresses to the aching breast tissue may also help alleviate these nippy ailments.

One solution is to cut a baby diaper in two, add a few drops of water onto each absorbent side until moist, and place both halves in the microwave for five seconds at a time until warm, but not burning hot. You don't want to scald those sensitive milkshakes.

Placing these quick compresses in your nursing bra can work wonders on over-worked breasts. Applying this same technique but placing the moist halves in a freezer instead until frozen may also offer relief.

Nipples can become quite sensitive from time to time. Changes in hormones, increased nipple activity, breastfeeding, various times during the menstrual cycle, sunburn, and stress can cause those chest circles to scream! Protection is important, so wear sunscreen if you're going nips-to-the-sky at the beach. When your nips cannot handle even a gentle brushing of clothing, breast shells offer a bit of a bubble buffer between your sensitive sets and your attire. Be gentle with your body, and yourself in general.

Loving your nipples means looking in the mirror and connecting the body to the mind. Sometimes, we do not like what we see. For some it can be more than superficial love handles or body hair we wish we could be rid of forever. These complaints are cosmetic.

What if in your mind and in your being, you are a twenty-three-year-old brunette man and you love books, horror films, working on cars, and dressing comfortably in jeans and a t-shirt. But then you pass a shiny store window and catch a glance at yourself and instead you see a twenty-three-year-old brunette woman with long hair and breasts where flatness should be. You're still you, but you don't look like you. It's alarming and this discrepancy can create insurmountable amounts of anxiety and depression and distress because what goes on inside the body doesn't match what everyone else sees outside.

We're talking about life as a transgender individual. It's not a mental health condition. Being transgender is a medical condition that requires hormone replacement therapy so the body can produce more of the missing hormone that will help individuals who have gender dysphoria reconcile who they are inside and out.

What does any of this have to do with nipples, you may be wondering. Everything!

When you look down at your dusty rose rib-apples, do they look feminine or are they more masculine? Excess breast tissue can mean all the difference between feeling comfortable in your own skin and seeking a surgeon to make the necessary cuts.

Finding a reputable surgeon who is trans-friendly and who will do your chest justice is such a difficult task that several trans individuals choose to live their lives in chest binders that ultimately warp their ribcages and thwart their ability to take in deep enough breaths. The circulatory system also suffers so the heart has to work harder to pump oxygenated blood throughout the body of a person who wears compression shirts to reshape themselves if they are to pass as who they authentically are in public without discrimination or worse.

Male-to-female (MTF) transitions require breast augmentation surgery similar to that of a woman who wishes to have larger breasts. The procedure is pretty straight forward with the same recovery time of about a week. Prior to surgery, months of estrogen hormone therapy initiate breast growth so that the skin is stretched to accommodate a fuller breast implant for a more appealing result. The nipples of the person undergoing surgery tend to lose their sensation with the introduction of these saline or silicone inserts.

It is female-to-male (FTM) transitions that are more difficult on the nipples because the areolas are cut away from the breast and set aside. After that, mammary glands, fatty breast tissue, skin and other structures are removed until a more flat chest is achieved. Sometimes pec implants (smaller versions of breast implants) are added but are not necessary. Lastly, drains are placed on both sides of the chest after the nipples are reshaped and replaced.

Sadly, these nipples also lose much of the sensation they had previously enjoyed and are much smaller versions of the same skin they used to be. Scars remain visible under the nipple area but generally fade over time especially if a vitamin E cream is applied daily.

Masculinizing chest surgery as discussed above, gender affirming surgery, and breast augmentation have the ability to save lives. When someone is misgendered, it steals a piece of themselves. Daily distress and discrimination can build until that person makes the most hopeless decision possible to remove themselves permanently and no amount of laws, prayer, or wishing can bring them back.

Being truly, unabashedly, who you are inside and out is a joy not everyone is free to enjoy. First, love yourself. Then love your neighbor. Live and let live has never applied more than in this case because love is love, and what does being male or being female have to do with anyone else but that person living their own life? The truth: it has nothing at all to do with you.

I'd like to throw one last point out for consideration; please hear me out: coconuts.

I would never fetishize, marginalize, demonize, or stigmatize trans-individuals ever. They're human beings the same as you or I. But you may be surprised to learn that singer Kim Petras, proud owner of her own set of 'Coconuts,' is in fact a transwoman. Look her up, her lyrics are fun and (sometimes) serious, upbeat, clever, and catchy.

She was born a male and has since become one of the most successful transgender artists of all time! She looks, sings, and uh… Behaves like a heterosexual female would in sexual situations (or so her lyrics would imply). It's not my business, so I'm not asking.

Take her song, 'Coconuts' as evidence. I offer for your viewing pleasure, 69 words from Ms. Petras about her "twins" and how confident she is in her new skin.

Kim Petras invites you to (2021):

> Look at these margarit-ta-tas! So juicy and so ripe, you wouldn't believe (believe). I give 'em different names, Cartier and Tiffany. I know you wanna bite, get your face in these (in these). I see 'em in your eyes, so meet the double D's: my coconuts! You can put 'em in your mouth (right now, right now, right now, right now). My coconuts! Watch 'em bounce up and down.

Witness the power of gender-affirming life changes that can save lives and create purpose in peoples' lives… Even if that purpose is to share some sexual liberation. As for Kim Petras, her sex is hers to sell and we're buying. Her message is no different than that of Kesha, Madonna, or Lady Gaga just because these artists kept the gender marker on their birth certificates the same as the day they were assigned it at birth. Sex is sex and being cisgender or transgender does not change this natural, normal part of being human. It also doesn't change the fact that changing one's nipples to match one's gender is okay, too. Between headlights and highbeams, whatever you dream you can be.

If you're taking them off, or putting them on, rearranging your nips to fit who you are can be more liberating than learning how to walk or getting your driver's license. Oh the places your nipples can go!

What makes a woman a woman is more than her nipples or bust size, the same as what makes a man a man has nothing to do with how flat his pecs may be. Society assigns stigma to certain nipples if they look more masculine or more feminine and gender affirming surgeries like those we discussed have the ability to remediate any discrepancies so that life can be lived unhidden and unburdened.

So let's make like a bra and be supportive of all our trans and nonbinary neigbors. We're all humans in it together and the world will be a much better place for it.

Being Body-positive in a Negative Society

Flaunt those identical eyesores! Make the most of your time on this planet by getting that nipple piercing (careful, this can decrease sensitivity!) or going braless even on the windiest of days. A chill may thrill your nips, but it's still all good. We're all for breaking barriers! Be bold and go beyond societal thresholds for modesty. You only live one life, but you live every second of every day…therefore, you should make every moment count. Being ashamed of how you were made does nothing to build you up, buttercup. So be beautifully you!

If it's summer, dress comfortably. When winter comes along and you still want the world to know you have cleavage, go for it! We're all for healthy self-expression.

Little known trivia for you while we're on the topic of warm or cold nipples: The same mechanism responsible for creating goosebumps, or piloerection, on the rest of the skin also plays a role in nipple erection. Furthermore, constant (THO, that's titty hard-on if you're not a teenage boy) or nipple rigidity is one unexpected side effect of getting one's nipples pierced. It's a party all the time and now everyone else will know it! Yikes. Don't let that deter your piercing plans, wear an undershirt or a padded bra and no one else will know that your maracas have transformed into bejeweled sombreros.

Which brings us right back to nipple piercings and the less permanent: nipple clamp.

Bedazzled (not vag-azzled…that's something completely different) boobies are all the rage. Aesthetically appetizing nip sprinkles could be just the boost your body modification quest is missing. Bring your A-game because this is going to hurt like a mother. Remember all those nerve endings and the colossal power nipple stim can have on an orgasm? All those sensitive connections come alive and start searing once the metal rod used in piercing begins to penetrate the areola.

Keep calm, pain is subjective and not everyone will feel it with the same level of intensity. The initial shock will wane to an ache and then will likely feel phenomenal after about six months-worth of healing and TLC. The opposite effect of nipple desensitization could also occur if nerve damage happens during the piercing process. Not to hamper your hooter parade but piercings are a serious commitment. We're giving you all the facts.

Piercing creates a fistula or healed hole in the flesh so you can expect an increased possibility of infection, swelling, or even body rejection. Sadly, no nipple is immune to nub-snub so make sure you're going to a reputable piercer who uses sterile tools to get the job done. Quality metals rather than nickel-plated ones for the actual jewelry are also a must for the bust. Stainless steel, gold, silver, and platinum are highly recommended.

Benefits of getting your nipples (one or both) pierced include possible heightened nipple sensation and changing those innie to outies. That's right! If you have either flat or inverted nipples, having them pierced may be able to correct this condition as the metal ends up elevating the breast flesh it runs through. Bonus: Breastfeeding is now an option (remember to remove any choking hazards before nursing sessions). Then you can resume wearing your 'bad,' totally rad raisin rods and go back to business as usual.

Can't commit to the long haul recovery or the permanence of creating a hole in your body? Try nipple clamps which can be worn as little, or as long, as you would like.

These less permanent playthings can be used during bedroom play or during the day for a slight tugging sensation that doesn't quit. Thin paperclip-looking attachments provide all the sensation you seek while being discreet. Office meetings have suddenly become much more bearable. Other options include more boisterous boob bondage and can be quite heavy.

To some, pain is pleasure and pleasure becomes more intense with an additional element of pain so there you are: clamps. Tweezer clamps look like a plastic set of tweezers mixed with a little BDSM, that's bondage, discipline/domination, sadism/submission, and masochism. Looking for more on those topics? You'll need another book for that because this one's about nipples.

To gauge how much or how little pain you'd like to mix with your pleasure, you (and your partner if you'd like) can experiment with flicking, licking, sucking, tweaking, twisting, pinching, and massaging the nipples, breasts, and arealoas to get a feel for what you like. Take turns! Reciprocity is so sexy.

It is recommended to warm the areola first with a little foreplay to make the skin more malleable. This also ensures less damage will be done to the area, if any. A cold nip is an unforgiving one. Next, you'll probably want to test the waters so to speak and place the 'teeth' of the teat clip further back on the nipple to test your pain threshold. A nip tip is much more sensitive than the base of the boob. Be prepared! Start slow because if you're going for temporary clampage, you don't want to do damage. You didn't want a piercing, remember?

After that, you can add weights a little at a time or remove or forego them as you wish. Twin nipple stim is all up to you so have fun and be as adventurous as you're comfortable being.

Whether you're a nipple clamps kind of person or a commited nipple piercer, either way, we know you're secret: Nip attention is your thing. And we love it! Honestly, creating adornments for your cherries brings out all the best in nipple play. If it's attention you seek, clamps and jewelry ensure that those discoballs are game for midnight dances and moves that will keep you stayin' alive all night.

Heading South But Staying Upbeat

Aging gracefully is an honor not bestowed upon everyone. If you're lucky enough to live a long life, congrats! You've accomplished something you should be proud of: Outliving the rest of your graduating class! Those losers should be so envious.

But as with anything else in life, getting older has its perks and its drawbacks. 'Perk' is not something that seems all that relevant anymore. What used to be pert and alert is now brushing your knees every time you step out of the shower.

We're talking nipples that used to point north and are now heading south for the winter. Menopause in females (when the ovaries no longer signal the production of estrogen and progesterone) and breakdown of skin elasticity with age can create an (im)perfect storm of sagging breasts. They spin in a whirlwind and sometimes suffocate you in your sleep; draping across you in wild array unless they're tied down using an over-the-shoulder boulder-holder like an anchor.

If your nips now brush the floor instead of pointing forward at attention, there are ways to care for this condition. We're here for support.

You may notice that nipple color tends to change with age for men and women alike. This is due, in part, because blood vessels become weaker over time. Carrying those heavy melanin basal cells through overworked, tired blood vessels means an increase in these heavy loads being dropped. This collection causes the areolas to become darker.

With age comes a few more deposits than increased melanin in certain areas: Fat also tends to collect in elderly individuals. It should be no surprise that the higher the body mass index (BMI), the larger the nipple.

And those blurry nurples tend to head south faster than a snowbird in September.

Dry skin could use a little moisturizer, so apply lotion generously on those mammaries and make sure you air dry completely before donning clothing. Wear a supportive bra or compression shirt to bed. One without an underwire or too much compression is best. Your days of getting poked in the middle of the night are probably already over.

Another unfortunate side effect of growing older is the formation of intraductal papilloma, or a growth behind the nipple tissue that is similar to a wart. Lactiferous duct ectasia due to mammary duct inflammation can be painful. The swollen, plugged milk ducts need medical treatment in order to obtain relief. This affliction mimics mastitis, a clogged milk duct, in breastfeeding mothers and can become serious quickly. So please, see a doctor if your nipples or surrounding tissues begin to ache and you have a fever.

Relief is in sight, and should never be embarrassing. Doctors have seen numerous conditions far worse than yours so whatever you need looked at is probably mild in comparison to what they've already seen before. They're professionals after all.

Our advice is always: When in doubt, get that checked out!

Conclusion

It's been nine chapters of nipples! That's included all nine varities of these sweet, supple sno-caps that wholly merit a whopping nine chapters just to cover the basics. We've come a long way from early nip development to voluptuous volcanoes and breast augmentation, to the low valley of breast cancer and the long road to recovery, and right back up north to the wonderland of nip lip color. It's been a wild ride full of peaks and valleys but we made it!

What have we learned from visiting the land of nipples? It is hoped that the answer is: a great deal! These tiny tornadoes have taken us on a whirlwind adventure through various cultures, intricate anatomy, and have offered a small sampling of evolutionary history shared across humanity.

We hope that you rest this nippy volume on your bookshelves, tuck it in tenderly between your other favorite books, and think of your adventure between book covers fondly. If you're ever in need of random nipple knowledge, know that we've got your back… and your front because this is a book about nipples.

When a Problem Comes Along, You Must Nip It!

What we can learn most by appreciating nipples is that at the end of the day, nipples don't care. If they're exposed, shrouded in mystery, or forgotten altogether (like at every boring work meeting), nipples face every issue the same way: without thought to who else cares. This is mainly due to their having no coherent intellectual thoughts of their own but that's merely a formality.

If everyone lived life to the fullest like a brandy set of nipples, the world would be a much less judgemental place. Life would be more enjoyable, more predictable. If you tweak a nipple, it will constrict. If you suck a lactating teat, it will let down. Cause and effect have more stability in the land of nipples. Every person on the planet would benefit from living life more freely… like a nipple.

The Life and Times of Nipple Ownership

It is imperative that you accept your nipples for what they are. It is equally important to appreciate others' nipples for what *they* are, as well. Every person possesses a purpose on this planet. And to be honest, no one is perfect. Airbrushed ideals plastered on pinup posters only serve unrealistic fantasies. The more realistic the expectation, the more satisfied in life you will become. That's not to knock the knockers that are enhanced by any means: To each their own! Know what you want and grab life by the bosom, metaphorically of course.

If we undress every prospective paramour expecting to see the same nips every time, that would get a bit boring… Unless, of course, we have chosen to marry those nips and commit for life! Even then, those nips are prone to change whether your partner is male, female, or any gender in between. Anyways, the point is to give grace to every nipple-owner. No pair of nips is the same but each should be given the same status all the same. Every nipple matters!

Glossary

Athelia: a medical condition, which may have underlying health causes, of being born without nipples

Alveoli: hollow cavities in breast tissue that contain milk-secreting cells

Breast Ptosis: a condition where breast tissue that had been taut begins to sag

Cisgender: when a person identifies as the sex they were assigned at birth, they are considered to be cisgender

Eutherian Mammal: a mammal (or lactating) animal that utilizes a placenta in utero to sustain the fetus during gestation

Endorphins: neurotransmitters naturally produced by the human brain; there are around 20 different types of these hormones, all of which reduce stress and pain

Feminism: the belief that every human should be given equality, equity, and opportunity in all aspects of life, primarily used in relation to socio-political and economic domains as well as basic human rights

Kallikrein: enzymes produced by the body that have the main function of breaking peptide bonds and directing other physiological processes

Letting Down (in breastfeeding): the term used to denote the moment nerves in the breast signal for the nipple to release milk in a nursing parent or other lactating animal

Mammal: a warm-blooded animal that grows hair, produces live young, and lactates to nourish their offspring

Mammary Gland: a collection of glands present in both males and females, but are further developed in females with the onset of puberty, that are responsible for milk production when signaled to do so by the presence of progesterone and prolactin

Mammary Ridge: this parallel line down both sides of an organism's ventral or front half of the body, from underarm to groin, and is mostly invisible in adults

Mammogram: an x-ray image of the breast used to check for abnormalities in breast tissues that help determine a possible diagnosis of breast cancer

Marsupial: a non-placental mammal that gives birth to live young and carries them through their most vulnerable developmental stage after birth, in a ventral pouch

Melanin: a genetically influenced substance made in the human body that determines the darkness and color of skin, eyes, and hair; also affected by how much direct sunlight a person's ancestors were exposed to during their lifetimes

Misogyny: dislike of, contempt for, or ingrained prejudice against women

Oxytocin: known as the "love hormone" this neurotransmitter is released during moments of pleasure, i.e. laughing, eating an enjoyable meal, during orgasm

Phytoestrogen: an estrogen-like compound that stimulates milk production when ingested

Piloerection: the technical term for goosebumps

Polythelia: a medical condition where a person is born with more than the usual set of two nipples or having supernumerary nipples; this may include having additional breast tissue supporting accessory nipple(s)

Prolactin: a hormone produced in the pituitary gland that is responsible for telling the mammary glands it is time to lactate

Supernumerary nipple: the presence of more than two distinct nipples, usually occurring along the milk line or mammary ridge

References

Anthony, J. (2016, August 24). Four ways you can legally bare your breasts in NYC. *Timeout.* https://www.timeout.com/newyork/blog/four-ways-you-can-legally-bare-your-breasts-in-nyc-082416#:~:text=Here's%20something%20you%20might%20not,New%20York%20City%20since%201992.

APA Dictionary of Psychology. (2022). Arousal. *American Psychological Association.* https://dictionary.apa.org/arousal

Barnes, Z. (2019, July 26). Your All-In-One Guide To Nipple Piercings. *Women'sHealth.* https://www.womenshealthmag.com/sex-and-love/a19912072/nipple-piercings/

Bonaguro, A. (2015, July 10). Why are women's nipples banned in public and on instagram, but men's nipples aren't? *Men's Health.* https://www.menshealth.com/sex-women/a19545146/nipple-double-standard/

Brooks, M. and Peiken, S. (1997). Bitch [Recorded by M. Brooks.] On *Blurring the Edges* [Album]. Capitol.

Campbell, N. (2018, March 8). Celebrities with a third nipple: Zac Efron, Lily Allen, and more! *Life and Style Mag.* https://www.lifeandstylemag.com/posts/celebrities-third-nipple-129253/

Castro, J. (2014). Can men lactate? *LiveScience.* https://www.livescience.com/45732-can-men-lactate.html

Celletti, E. N. (2018, April 10). Your guide to breast augmentation, from cost to recovery time. *Allure.*

https://www.allure.com/story/breast-augmentation-everything-you-need-to-know

Charo. (2003). The Surreal Life (TV Series 2003). *IMDB.com*. Retrieved from https://www.imdb.com/title/tt0337784/characters/nm0004819

Cohen, D. (2001). Cultural variation: Considerations and implications. *Psychological Bulletin, 127,* 451-471. https://www.researchgate.net/profile/Dov-Cohen-5/publication/11900913_Cultural_variation_Considerations_and_implications/links/58f40acea6fdcc11e569f373/Cultural-variation-Considerations-and-implications.pdf

Endorphins: The brain's natural pain reliever. (2021, July 20). *Harvard Health Publishing.* https://www.health.harvard.edu/mind-and-mood/endorphins-the-brains-natural-pain-reliever

Gonzalez, F., Brown, F. E., Gold, M. E., Walton, R. L., Shafer, B. (1993, October). Preoperative and postoperative nipple-areola sensibility in patients undergoing reduction mammaplasty. *Plast Reconstr Surg.* 92(5):809-14.

Hazlewood, L. (1966). These boots are made for walkin' [Recorded by N. Sinatra]. On *Boots* [Album]. Reprise Records.

Heine, S. J. (2016). *Cultural Psychology.* Brantford, Ont., W. Ross Macdonald School Resource Services Library, 2017.

The Incredible Milk-Producing Male Bat (n.d.). *Bats Magazine.* vol. 13, no. 1. https://www.batcon.org/article/the-incredible-milk-producing-male-bat/

Jacobs, J. (2019, November 22). Will Instagram ever 'free the nipple'? *New York Times.* https://www.nytimes.com/2019/11/22/arts/design/instagram-free-the-nipple.html

Kayhart, K. (2021, November 21). Janet Jackson and Justin Timberlake's 'Nipplegate' controversy the focus of new documentary that reveals tale of two aftermaths for the pop stars. *DailyMail.* https://www.dailymail.co.uk/tvshowbiz/article-10226103/Janet-Jackson-Justin-Timberlakes-Nipplegate-controversy-focus-new-documentary.html

Kelly, A. J., Dubbs, S. L., Barlow, F. K., Zietsch, B. P. (2018). Male and female nipples as a test case for the assumption that functional features vary less than nonfunctional byproducts. *Adaptive Human Behavior and Physiology.*

Kinonen, S. (2017, May 9). Your perfect nude lipstick is the color of your nipples — But there's a catch. *Allure.* https://www.allure.com/story/nipples-match-nude-lipstick-shade

Komisaruk, B. R., Wise, N, Frangos, E., Liu, W-C., Allen, K., and Brody, S. (2011, October 1). Women's clitoris, vagina and cervix mapped on the sensory cortex: fMRI evidence. *J Sex Med* 2011;8:2822–2830. https://doi.org/10.1111/j.1743-6109.2011.02388.x

LaPorte, K. (2019, October). Lingerie by the decade - 1940's. *Bobbins & Bombshells.* https://www.bobbinsandbombshells.com/blog/2016/10/19/fashionable-history-lingerie-by-decade-1940s

The Let-Down - Breastmilk - Every Ounce Counts. (2022). Texas WIC. https://www.breastmilkcounts.com/breastfeeding-101/the-let-down/

Levin, R., and Meston, C. (2006). Nipple/Breast stimulation and sexual arousal in young men and women. *J Sex Med.* 2006 May;3(3):450-4. https://pubmed.ncbi.nlm.nih.gov/16681470/

Love, S. M., and Barsky, S. H. (2004). Anatomy of the nipple and breast ducts revisited. Cancer, 101:1947-1957. https://doi.org/10.1002/cncr.20559

MacGuill, D. (2018, October 5). Did president Donald Trump allow the violence against women act to expire? *Snopes.*

https://www.snopes.com/fact-check/trump-violence-against-women-act/

Male and Female Breast Anatomy. (n.d.). *Dreamstime.* https://www.dreamstime.com/stock-images-male-female-breast-anatomy-image12436234

Mammary gland anatomy function & diagram. (2018, January 20). *Healthline.* https://www.healthline.com/human-body-maps/mammary-gland#1

Mayer, J. (2001). Your body is a wonderland [Recorded by J. Mayer]. On *Room for Squares* [Album]. Columbia Aware.

Melanin: What is it, types and benefits. (2022, March 29). *Cleveland Clinic.* https://my.clevelandclinic.org/health/body/22615-melanin

Onwurah, N. (Director), & Gardner, L. (Producer). (1993). Monday's Girls [Video file]. British Broadcasting Corporation. Retrieved from Academic Video Online: Premium database.

Park, C. S. and G. L. Lindberg. 2004. The mammary gland and lactation. pp. 720-741 in *Dukes' Physiology of Domestic Animals*, W.O. Reece, ed. (Publisher not identified.)

Peralta, E. (2015, August 24). Topless in New York: The court case that makes going top free legal. *NPR.* https://www.npr.org/sections/thetwo-way/2015/08/24/434315957/topless-in-new-york-the-legal-case-that-makes-going-top-free-legal-ish

Platypus. (n.d.). *American Museum of Natural History.* https://www.amnh.org/exhibitions/extreme-mammals/meet-your-relatives/platypus#:~:text=Like%20all%20mammals%2C%20 monotreme%20mothers,it%20from%20tufts%20of%20fur.

Pop, J. (1999). The bad touch [Recorded by Bloodhound Gang]. On *Hooray for Boobies* [Album]. Geffen.

Robinson, G. W. 2007. Cooperation of signaling pathways in embryonic mammary gland development. *Nature Reviews Genetics*, 8: 963-972. https://www.nature.com/articles/nrg2227

Robinson, J. E., and Short R. V. (1977, May 7). *Changes in breast sensitivity at puberty*, during the menstrual cycle, and at parturition. https://pubmed.ncbi.nlm.nih.gov/861531/

Rubinstein, C. (2021, December 29). Breast augmentation size chart – implant sizes and cup sizes. https://drcraigrubinstein.com.au/blogs/breast-augmentation-size-chart-implant-sizes-and-cup-sizes/

Sauter, et al., (2002). Ethnic variation in Kallikrein expression in nipple aspirate fluid, *IJC*, 100(6).

Skandalakis, J. E., Skandalakis, P. N., Weidman, T. A., Skandalakis, L. J. Breast. In: *Skandalakis' Surgical Anatomy*, Skandalakis, J. E., Weidman, T. A., Foster, R. S. Jr, et al (Eds), McGraw Hill, New York 2004.

Smith, D. (2005, October 10). Marsupial mammals. *Berkeley.* https://ucmp.berkeley.edu/mammal/marsupial/marsupial.html

Sullivan, N. and Levitas, J. (2021, December 8). Modern western culture & social life. https://study.com/academy/lesson/modern-western-culture-social-life.html

Taylor, M. S. (2014, August 27). *Anatomy - Do male mammals other than humans have nipples?*

https://biology.stackexchange.com/questions/3834/do-male-mammals-other-than-humans-have-nipples

There are 8 types of nipples in the world. (2022, June 10). *Newfashion.* https://www.life-stylez.com/article/there-are-8-types-of-nipples-in-the-world,3338.html

Timberlake, J. (2002). Rock your body [Recorded by J. Timberlake]. On *Justified* [Album]. Jive.

Top surgery for transgender men and nonbinary people (n.d.) *Mayo Clinic.* https://www.mayoclinic.org/tests-procedures/top-surgery-for-transgender-men/about/pac-20469462

Topfreedom. (n.d.). *Bionity.* https://www.bionity.com/en/encyclopedia/Topfreedom.html

Tunell, A. (2017, May 10). We matched our lipstick to our nipples & things got interesting. *Refinery29.* https://www.refinery29.com/en-us/2017/05/153857/real-women-nipples-nude-lipstick-colors

Tunell, A. (2017, July 1). We wore "vagina lipstick" — & it made everyone uncomfortable. *Yahoo.com.* https://www.yahoo.com/lifestyle/wore-vagina-lipstick-made-everyone-203500207.html

2010 : Geraldine Hoff Doyle, the real-life model for we can do it Rosie the riveter, dies in Lansing (2018-12-26). (2018, December 26). *Michigan Day by Day.* http://harris23.msu.domains/event/2010-

geraldine-hoff-doyle-the-real-life-model-for-we-can-do-it-rosie-the-riveter-dies-in-lansing/

Valdes, R., Ogren, R., Oliver, V. R., Lil Aaron, Aguilar, A. J., De Saint Rome, C., and Gottwald, L. (2021) Coconuts [Recorded by K. Petras]. On *Coconuts* [Album]. Republic.

Veltmaat, J. (2012, April 12). Welcome to the laboratory of mammary gland development. http://www.veltmaatlab.net/research.html

Watson, C. J., and W. T. Khaled. 2008. Mammary development in the embryo and adult: a journey of morphogenesis and commitment. Development 135: 995-1003.

Watson, S. (2018, March 13). No nipples (Athelia): Cause, treatment, complications. *Heathline.* https://www.healthline.com/health/no-nipples

Weiss, R. E. (2021, June 20). What are Montgomery's Tubercles? *Very Well Family.* https://www.verywellfamily.com/montgomerys-tubercles-2759956#:~:text=Montgomery's%20tubercles%20serve%20their%20greatest,your%20baby%20from%20certain%20infections

What is breast cancer screening? (2021, September 22). *CDC.* https://www.cdc.gov/cancer/breast/basic_info/screening.htm

Women's March (2022). Summer of rage. *Women's March.* https://www.womensmarch.com/

Zucca-Matthes, G., Urban, C., & Vallejo, A. (2016). Anatomy of the nipple and breast ducts. *Gland Surgery*, 5(1), 326–336. https://gs.amegroups.com/article/view/7703/9415